Traumatic Brain Injury in Children and Adolescents

Traumatic Brain Injury in Children and Adolescents

A SOURCEBOOK FOR TEACHERS AND OTHER SCHOOL PERSONNEL

MARY P. MIRA
BONNIE FOSTER TUCKER
JANET SIANTZ TYLER

pro·ed

8700 Shoal Creek Boulevard
Austin, Texas 78757

The authors, whose names are listed alphabetically, have the following affiliations:

Mary P. Mira, The Children's Rehabilitation Unit, the University of Kansas Medical Center, Kansas City, KS.

Bonnie Foster Tucker, Head Injury Association of Kansas and Greater Kansas City, Shawnee Mission, KS.

Janet Siantz Tyler, Department of Special Education, the University of Kansas Medical Center, Kansas City, KS.

© 1992 by PRO-ED, Inc.

All rights reserved. No part of this book may be reproduced in any form or by any means without the prior written permission of the publisher.

Printed in the United States of America

Library of Congress Cataloging-in-Publication Data

Mira, Mary P.
　　Traumatic brain injury in children and adolescents : sourcebook for teachers and other school personnel / Mary P. Mira, Bonnie Foster Tucker, Janet Siantz Tyler.
　　　　p.　　cm.
　　Includes bibliographical references.
　　ISBN 0-89079-531-2
　　1. Brain-damaged children—Rehabilitation.　2. Brain—Wounds and injuries—Patients—Rehabilitation.　3. Brain damage—Complications and sequelae.　4. Brain-damaged children—Education.
　　5. Mainstreaming in education.　I. Tucker, Bonnie Foster.
　　II. Tyler, Janet Siantz.　III. Title.
　　[DNLM: 1. Brain Injuries—in adolescence.　2. Brain Injuries—in infancy & childhood.　3. Brain Injuries—rehabilitation.
　　4. Education, Special.　WS 340 M671t]
　　RJ496.B7M57　1992
　　617.4′81044′083—dc20
　　DNLM/DLC
　　for Library of Congress　　　　　　　　　　　　　　　　92-3454
　　　　　　　　　　　　　　　　　　　　　　　　　　　　　　　　CIP

pro·ed

8700 Shoal Creek Boulevard
Austin, Texas 78757

3　4　5　6　7　8　9　10　　98　97　96

Contents

Foreword / ix

Preface / xi

Acknowledgments / xiii

1 Introduction / 1

2 Facts About Traumatic Brain Injury in Children and Adolescents / 3
INCIDENCE OF TBI AMONG CHILDREN / 3
SEVERITY OF TBI / 5
CAUSES OF TBI / 6
RISK FACTORS IN TBI / 6

3 Developmental Aspects of Traumatic Brain Injury / 9
ONGOING BRAIN DEVELOPMENT / 9
INFLUENCE OF AGE / 10
DISRUPTION OF SOCIAL DEVELOPMENT / 10

4 *Physical Effects of Traumatic Brain Injury* / 13
NEUROPATHOLOGY OF TBI / 13
CHARACTERISTICS OF AN INJURED BRAIN / 14
INITIAL EFFECTS OF INJURY: THE EARLY ACUTE PHASE / 15
PERSISTING EFFECTS OF TBI / 18
INTERACTION OF PROBLEMS RESULTING FROM TBI / 24

5 *Psychosocial Effects of Traumatic Brain Injury* / 27
TYPES OF PSYCHOSOCIAL PROBLEMS / 27
AGE CONSIDERATIONS / 29
ISSUES IN ADOLESCENT TBI / 29
THE SCHOOL'S ROLE IN PSYCHOSOCIAL OUTCOME / 31

6 *Continuum of Treatment for Traumatic Brain Injury* / 35
COMPONENTS OF A COMPREHENSIVE PROGRAM / 35
HOW SCHOOLS CAN INTERACT WITH HOSPITALS / 38
ISSUES IN FINANCING THE REHABILITATION/
  RECOVERY PROGRAM / 40

7 *Planning for School Reentry* / 43
FRAMEWORK FOR DEVELOPING AN EDUCATIONAL PLAN
  FOLLOWING A TBI / 43
ESTABLISHING COMMUNICATION BETWEEN REHABILITATION
  PROFESSIONALS AND SCHOOLS / 43
APPROPRIATE EDUCATIONAL GOALS FOR STUDENTS
  WITH TBI / 44
CRITICAL ELEMENTS THAT SHOULD BE IN PLACE
  IN SCHOOLS / 45
BARRIERS THAT CAN IMPEDE SUCCESSFUL
  SCHOOL REINTEGRATION / 46
HOSPITAL-TO-SCHOOL TRANSITION PLANNING / 47
EVALUATING AND MODIFYING THE SCHOOL ENVIRONMENT / 51
SCHOOL CALENDAR AND DAILY SCHEDULING / 52
IEP PLANNING / 53
CASE MANAGEMENT / 54

8 *Assessment of the Student with Traumatic Brain Injury* / 59
LONGITUDINAL NATURE OF ASSESSMENT / 59
IMPORTANCE OF A NEUROPSYCHOLOGICAL EXAMINATION / 60
COMPONENTS OF A NEUROPSYCHOLOGICAL EVALUATION / 61

DIFFERENCES BETWEEN NEUROPSYCHOLOGICAL
  AND OTHER EVALUATIONS / 62
NEUROPSYCHOLOGICAL BATTERIES / 63
UNDERSTANDING NEUROPSYCHOLOGICAL FINDINGS / 65
IMPLICATIONS OF NEUROPSYCHOLOGICAL DEFICITS
  FOR CLASSROOM FUNCTIONING / 65

9 *Programming for Students with Traumatic Brain Injury* / 69
COGNITIVE RETRAINING WITHIN THE SCHOOL / 69
THE EDUCATOR'S ROLE IN COGNITIVE RETRAINING / 70
PROGRAMMING FOR SPECIFIC DEFICITS / 71
DEALING WITH BEHAVIOR PROBLEMS / 76
TEACHER REACTIONS TO THE LONG-TERM EFFECTS OF TBI / 77
SOURCES OF TEACHER FRUSTRATION / 78
COMMUNITY RESPONSES TO LONG-STANDING EFFECTS / 79
THE SCHOOL'S ROLE IN STUDENT'S CAREER/LIFE PLANNING / 79

10 *Families of Children and Adolescents
with Traumatic Brain Injury* / 83
EMOTIONAL REACTIONS OF THE FAMILY / 83
SOURCES OF FAMILY DISTRESS / 86
HOW SCHOOLS CAN WORK WITH FAMILIES OF CHILDREN
  WITH TBI / 89

11 *Summary and Implications for Future Directions* / 91
EFFECTS OF TBI / 91
REENTRY TO SCHOOL / 93
TEACHING THE STUDENT WITH TBI / 94
EMERGING ISSUES / 95
PREVENTION / 96

APPENDIX A: *Bibliography* / 97

APPENDIX B: *Physical Facilities and Planning Checklist for Schools* / 101

APPENDIX C: *Checklist for School Reentry* / 105

APPENDIX D: *Evaluation Summary* / 109

APPENDIX E: *Neuropsychological Report* / 117

GLOSSARY / 125

REFERENCES / 129

INDEX / 131

FOREWORD

This book grew out of our experiences in assisting students with traumatic brain injuries (TBI) to reenter school successfully. We realized early on that several things could be done to improve a student's chances for school success following such an injury.

We recognized that our own training in special education and psychology, although generally considered comprehensive and thorough, had not addressed needs of the group of children surviving TBI. Because school is the place where most of the children go after their injuries have healed, we knew that teachers—both regular and special—needed training in effectively meeting the needs of students with TBI. We found that all too often educators waited for these children to be dismissed from the hospital before attempting any educational planning or intervention.

We have observed problems arising because continuity between hospital and school was lacking, so we try in this book to assist educators in assuming an active role during the period of hospitalization. We advocate developing a service continuum whereby gaps between hospital recommendations and school realities are understood and acceptable to all concerned. Bringing educators into the hospital for staffings, family planning meetings, and therapy sessions generate benefits for both hospital and school professionals, but it especially benefits the student.

Because we are based in a hospital, we benefited from seeing these students as patients. We observed progress from coma through rehabilitation therapies to discharge. As we worked with educators, we conveyed significant information about the children's needs in a unique way.

We suggest that schools establish a practice of designating a school case manager to initiate hospital–school communication and to interpret information unique to each. We also suggest early and regular hospital–school contact to forestall potential education disruptions. This information is incorporated into this book, which provides readers with professional approaches to school intervention for students with TBI.

PREFACE

This book is about students with traumatic brain injury (TBI), from preschoolers through adolescents. We focus particularly on students whose injuries were moderate to severe—that is, those expected to suffer educationally significant *residual* (lasting) impairments. Our purpose is to provide an introduction to the characteristics and needs of children and adolescents with TBI as they present to schools.

In this book, we translate significant medical information into language useful to educators. We include practical suggestions, characteristics, short- and long-term effects of TBI, development of comprehensive programs, and planning for successful school maintenance. We have drawn from our experiences developing programs for students, as well as the body of information developed in recent years.

The book is designed for school professionals whose responsibilities include serving individuals with disabilities. This includes not only special educators and regular teaching staff, but diagnostic team members and those who provide special services to children with disabilities in schools. The identification of TBI as a categorical disability (Individuals with Disabilities Education Act, 1990) is too recent to have affected how students with TBI are educated. They are being served in the entire range of categorical special education programs.

Those who have significant disabilities may be in programs for physically impaired, mentally retarded, or severely multihandicapped. Those with milder injuries and residuals may be served by programs for students with behavior disorders or learning disabilities. School professionals in all of these settings have a need to know more about children with TBI.

ACKNOWLEDGMENTS

Professionals whose pioneering efforts and conceptualizations have significantly shaped the direction of our work include Ron Savage, Mark Ylvisaker, Byron Rourke, and Ellen Lehr. Their works and other materials useful for educators are in the annotated bibliography (Appendix A) and the reference list.

We are also indebted to the students, families, and school professionals who have participated in planning and developing educational programs especially suited to the altered educational needs that head injuries produce. Their willingness to learn new instructional techniques, adapt existing programs, and advocate for sound educational goals and management have provided models for others to emulate.

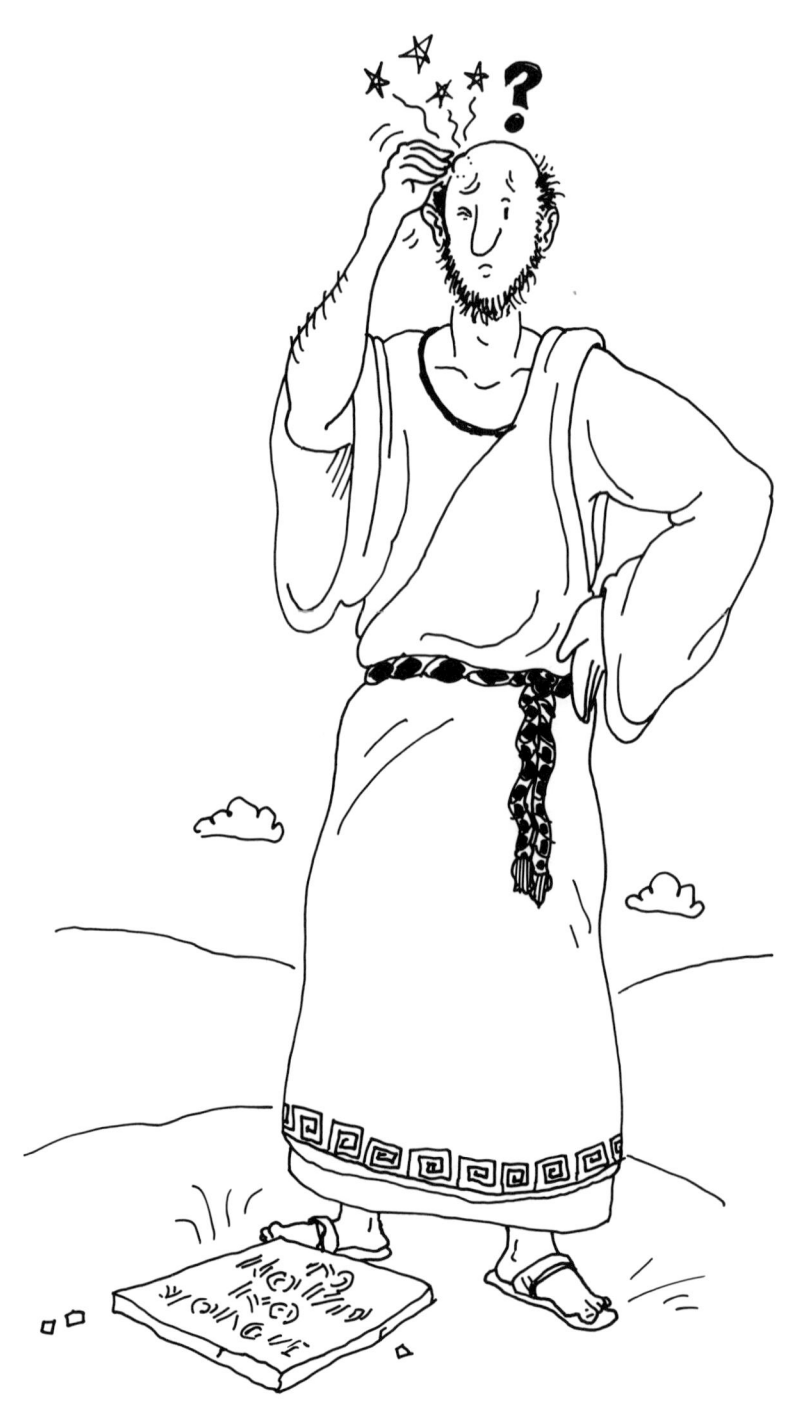

1

Introduction

The Individuals with Disabilities Education Act of 1990, an amendment of the 1975 Education for all Handicapped Children Act (Public Law [PL] 94-142), has created a category for serving individuals with traumatic brain injury (TBI). In recommending this legislation, the committee noted the lack of a specific definition, reporting method, and consistent manner of identifying this population. Creating a category for students with TBI therefore represents a major step toward identifying needs and requirements for education and related services. It will also facilitate personnel training and program planning.

A traumatic brain injury is "an insult to the brain caused by an external force that may produce diminished or altered states of consciousness, which results in impaired cognitive abilities or physical functioning" (National Head Injury Foundation, 1989, p. 2). It can also result in the disturbance of behavioral or emotional functioning. A traumatic brain injury may occur when there is a blow to the head or when the head slams against a stationary object. Such injuries happen in car accidents when the head hits the windshield or in bicycle accidents when the head hits the ground. The brain may also be injured by penetration of foreign objects, such as bullets or lawn darts.

The brain controls all the body's actions and functions, including digestion, temperature, breathing, heartbeat, and blood pressure.

It receives and interprets messages from the sense organs and directs the body to respond or move or react to the environment. If injured, the brain affects the body's systems in unpredictable ways. Although the student may appear normal, cognitive deficits always follow a severe head injury and usually follow a moderate injury. Traumatic brain injury induces permanent changes.

TBI is now gaining the attention of educators as a new disability; however, people have been fascinated with the effects of brain injury throughout history. A case documented in 30 A.D. by Maximus described a man's loss of memory for letters after a blow to the head. Several 19th-century researchers studied language disorders following trauma to the brain. Scientists at that time also studied written language and perceptual motor problems following TBI (Wiederholt, 1974).

Because TBI usually affects academic performance significantly, special education services are often needed for the student's ongoing education and rehabilitation. As a result, special education resources, such as multidisciplinary evaluations, parental involvement, and development of an Individualized Educational Plan (IEP), become important considerations. Although the special education system offers the necessary structure to meet the needs of students with TBI, it currently lacks knowledgeable staff and special programmatic features for students with TBI whose characteristics do not readily match existing categories.

As a result, students with TBI have been served in programs for children with other health impairments, although the former are often more capable physically than the latter. Some have been served in learning disabilities programs because of their attention and organization deficits. However, students with TBI differ from children with learning disabilities because they demonstrate greater discrepancies between abilities, make more uneven progress, and generally require a more cognitive than academic focus. Furthermore, they do not resemble students with mental retardation, with whom some also have been placed, because they tend to retain distinct islands of skills, and their learning does not resemble the slow, steady pace of students with developmental disabilities. Thus, the expansion of the special education mandate to include students with TBI represents a major event and promises to result in more appropriate educational programming for these students.

2

Facts About Traumatic Brain Injury in Children and Adolescents

Incidence of TBI Among Children

Traumatic brain injury is not a rare occurrence among children. Thus, it is surprising that it has received so little attention by educators. Approximately 1 in 500 children is hospitalized with a head injury each year, and 1 in 30 (3%) children born this year will sustain a head injury before late adolescence (Annegers, 1983). Because the effects of TBI may persist for years, the cumulative number of children who are struggling in school with the residuals of injury to the brain is larger than 3%. For educators, these statistics mean that a small school district can anticipate having several children who have suffered a significant injury to the brain. Large districts will have over 100 such students.

The peak incidence of TBI for the population as a whole falls between the ages 15 and 24; however, it is almost as common among younger children (Kraus, 1987). After the first year of life, boys who

4 *Traumatic Brain Injury in Children and Adolescents*

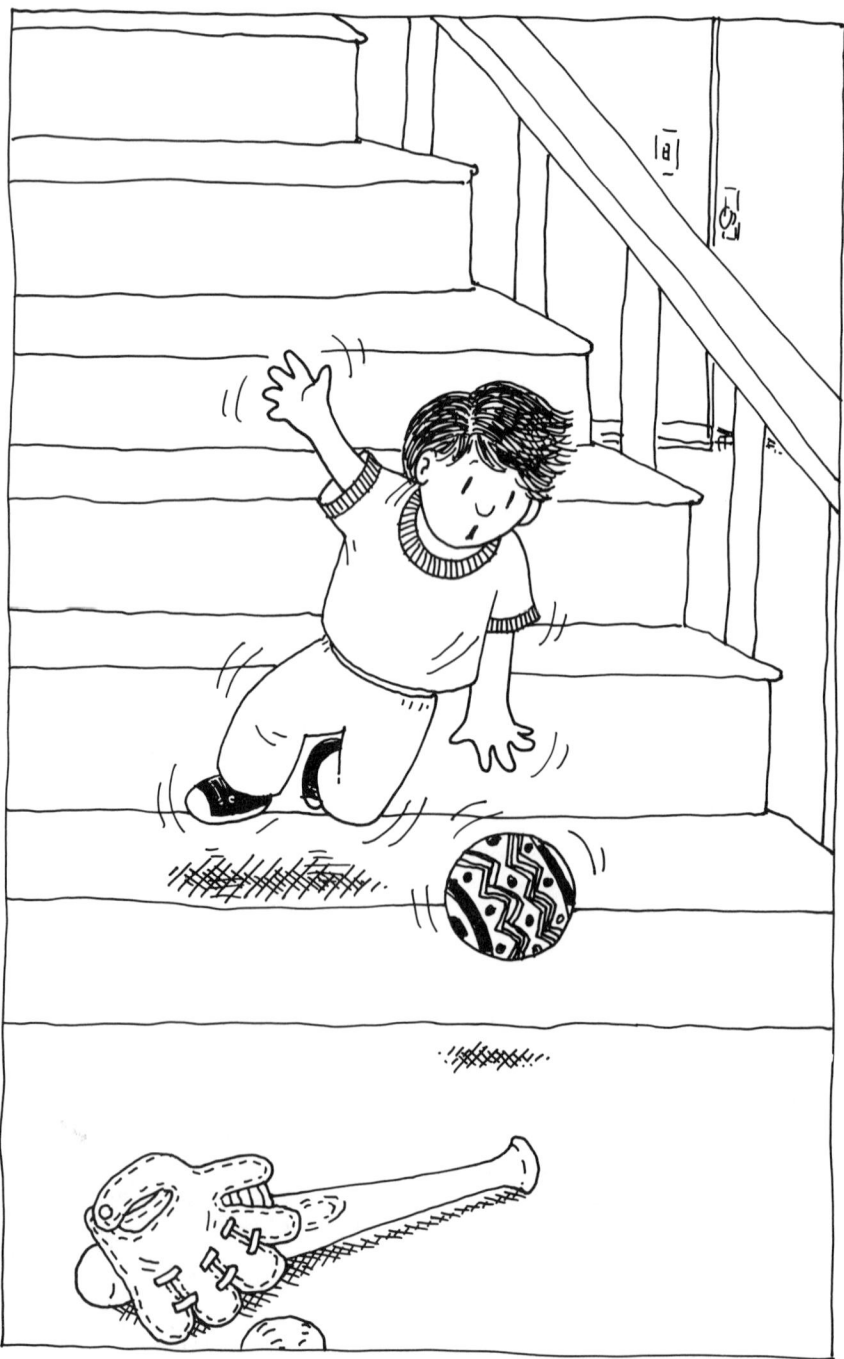

are injured outnumber girls two to one. Of children who are hospitalized, approximately 15% have moderate to severe injuries that will have long-term effects on learning and behavior. Even some of the children sustaining mild injuries with no loss of consciousness may demonstrate behavioral or cognitive residuals.

We do not have a clear picture of incidence trends among children. Use of helmets, particularly for motorcyclists, has reduced the rate of deaths and severe brain injury; seat belt use has also reduced deaths from severe injury. On the other hand, improvements in emergency evacuation and trauma care, even in rural areas, and neurosurgical advances now enable more severely injured children, who previously would have died, to survive.

Severity of TBI

It is important for educators to be told about the severity of a student's TBI because that information provides some clues about anticipated long-term outcome. Injury severity is based on the amount and type of damage to the skull and brain, and the level of consciousness after the injury. No standardized system has been developed for classifying severity of brain injury. The following grouping of mild, moderate, and severe injuries is based on a compilation from several sources.

Mild brain injuries show signs of a *concussion* or a blow resulting in some aftereffects, such as dizziness or loss of consciousness, for less than an hour. There is no skull fracture. The majority of brain injuries are mild. In the past, it was felt that mildly injured children would suffer no residual impairments and would quickly pick up their school activities and learning again. We now recognize, however, that there are, in fact, both neurological and cognitive–behavioral effects of mild injury, including diffuse changes within the brain. Also, memory and attention problems may persist. If not recognized as residuals of the injury and dealt with, these problems may lead to long-term academic or behavioral difficulties.

People who experience *moderate* brain injuries lose consciousness from 1 to 24 hours or have a skull fracture. Children with moderate TBI may develop secondary neurological problems, such as swelling within the brain and subsequent complications. Also, many of these children may require neurosurgery. They may show medical as well as cognitive *sequelae* or consequences, which may persist for some time.

In *severe* brain injuries, people experience loss of consciousness for more than 24 hours, or evidence of *contusion* (actual bruising of brain tissue) or *intracranial hematoma* (bleeding within the brain). These children's condition is so critical that they will be cared for in the intensive care unit of a hospital. Upon regaining consciousness, they will demonstrate motor, language, and cognitive problems. They will generally have lifelong cognitive deficits that will influence subsequent learning.

Causes of TBI

Motor vehicle accidents (in which the child is a passenger, pedestrian, or bicyclist), falls, and abuse represent the primary causes of children's head injuries. Among children under 5 years of age, falls are the most common cause, with the peak incidence occurring below age 2. In this below–school-age group, accidents as passengers in motor vehicles is the second highest cause. Physical abuse is a significant cause among infants and toddlers. Indeed, the true incidence of abuse-induced TBI may be greater than reported, and may be one of the most common causes in the very young. Three-fourths of infant and toddler head injuries occur in the home because both abuse and falls often occur here.

Younger school-age children are most often injured in pedestrian– or bicycle–vehicular accidents, and as passengers. With age, trauma stemming from recreation and sports injuries increases. Finally, among adolescents, predominant causes are motor vehicle accidents, sports injuries, and, in some populations, assaults.

The severity of TBI also varies with age. Abuse-related injuries among infants (at least those that are diagnosed) are often severe. For example, when the abuse takes the form of vigorous shaking of the infant, associated damage often results, such as hemorrhages in the retina that result in visual problems. Injuries from falls are generally more severe in infants than in toddlers or older children. This is because infants generally fall from greater heights, such as from a parent's arms or off furniture, whereas toddlers topple over when walking.

Risk Factors in TBI

Children's cognitive and behavioral characteristics before the trauma play a role in risk of injury. Children who sustain traumatic brain injuries, particularly mild ones, are generally reported to have a higher incidence of prior behavior problems. Overactive and impulsive children may take greater risks than others and, therefore, engage in more dangerous activities leading to injury.

Other risk factors are related to the child's environment. Children who sustain brain injuries often come from families that are experiencing stress. These families tend to have a higher than average incidence of marital instability and economic problems. Environmental variables associated with abuse-induced TBI include crowding, family instability, and high stress.

One TBI increases the risk of another injury to the brain for a variety of reasons, including impulsiveness and judgment deficits, as well as balance and coordination problems resulting from the first injury. The child's age is another influence. Children below age 15 who experienced one TBI are twice as likely to sustain another TBI than children in general, and those over age 15 are three times as likely.

Summary

Severity of Injury

- Mild—loss of consciousness less than 1 hour
- Moderate—loss of consciousness between 1 and 24 hours
- Severe—loss of consciousness more than 24 hours

Causes of TBI

- Motor vehicle accidents
- Falls
- Abuse
- Sports injuries
- Assault

Risk Factors

- Prior behavior problems
- Family stress
- Family instability
- Crowded living conditions
- Prior TBI

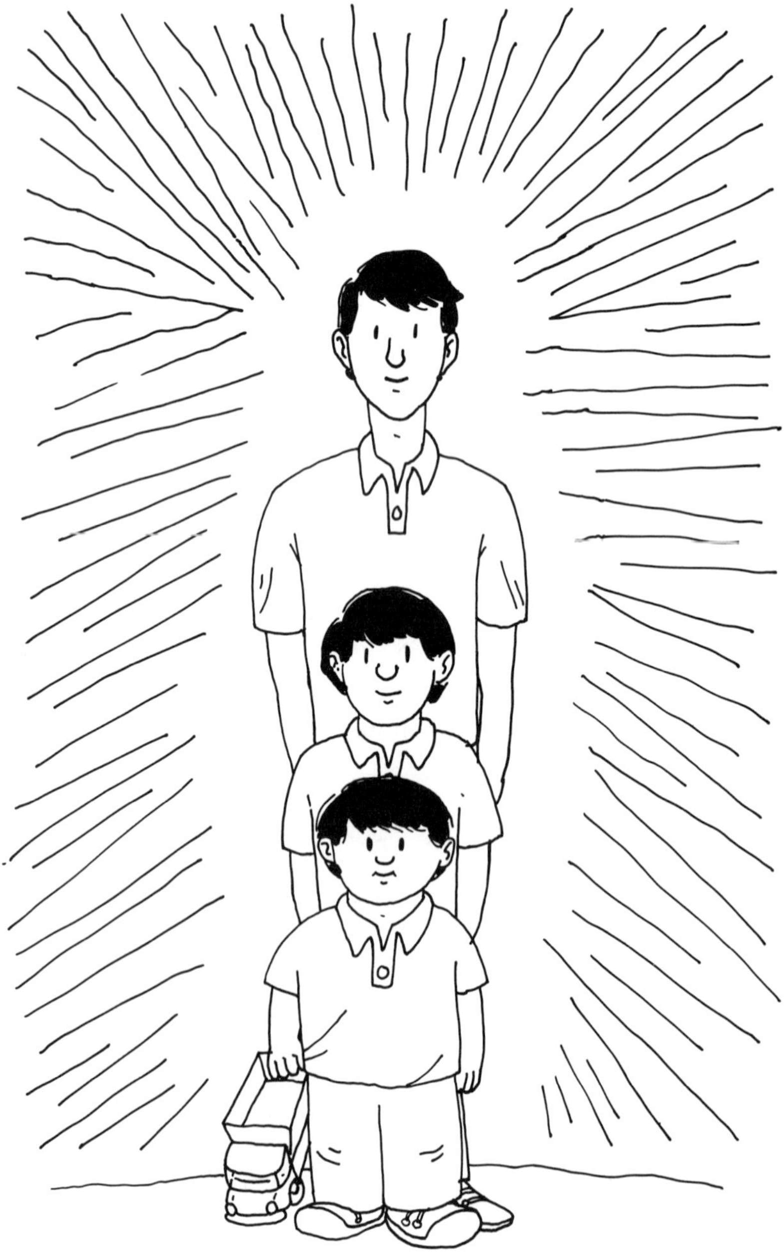

3

Developmental Aspects of Traumatic Brain Injury

To appreciate the profound effects of TBI in children, we must keep in mind that such an injury occurs to a developing brain; that is, the course of recovery is superimposed on the child's normal development, in contrast to the recovery process of an injured adult, whose brain is mature. Therefore, knowledge about TBI recovery derived from adults may not be true for children. Also, in planning for the child, we must consider the previous developmental pattern.

Even when educators have access to developmental histories, prediction and planning are difficult because the child's subsequent developmental pattern may be unpredictable. An injury to the brain may affect future development in several ways. It may (a) change the course and rate of development, (b) reduce the ultimate level of achievement of skills, (c) wipe out previously attained skills, and (d) affect the development of skills that have not yet emerged at the time of the injury.

Ongoing Brain Development

The brain does not stop developing in infancy, but continues to develop over a greater time span than generally recognized. For example, growth of cellular structure is ongoing during the first 2 years of life. Some connections between the sensory systems that are vital for academic learning do not mature until the early elementary school years. Changes in the organization and interconnection of brain systems and in the maturation of the nerve fibers continue at least through adolescence. Similarly, some of the brain systems involved in higher level cognitive activities, such as judgment and planning, do not mature until at least the late elementary school years. For these reasons, a TBI occurring even as late as adolescence will affect a brain that is still changing.

Influence of Age

The results of a TBI are not so straightforward that we can pronounce that their effects are greater or less at any age. Therefore, the widespread notion that younger children recover more successfully from head injury than older children or adults is incorrect. The evidence is that children have greater lifelong problems following TBI than do adults, because TBI has the most profound effect on incompletely developed skills. Young children possess fewer well-entrenched, automatic skills and a smaller knowledge base upon which to build recovery. Infants and toddlers under age 2 suffer greater effects from TBI than do older children. The injury to the brain alters the ways in which a child perceives and processes stimuli and interacts with the environment. Because the major impact of TBI involves the ability to acquire new learning, the younger child will be more disadvantaged.

Injuries that occur before children enter school present special problems for educators. In many cases, school personnel are not informed about the injury when the child is enrolled. Thus, teachers cannot anticipate and prepare for later learning problems. Although young children may appear to be doing well cognitively after a TBI, they may demonstrate deficits in attention and other foundational cognitive skills, resulting in academic difficulties in the early grades. Because it is important for educators to be aware of an early history of TBI, a question about it should be a part of all routine school entry procedures.

Disruption of Social Development

Injuries to infants and toddlers present special problems for families. This is the time when children are viewed as most vulnerable, in need of care, and not responsible for their own safety. Therefore, an injury at this age raises questions about who was responsible for the accident and how it could have been prevented if someone had behaved differently.

In the preschool years, although dependent on adults for care, children begin to participate in their care. An accident that even temporarily disrupts a child's ability to care for his or her needs alters the progress toward independence and may have a lifelong impact on the development of self-determination.

The early school years are a time of important social development as children interact more with others outside the home. A TBI at this period can disrupt emerging social relationships. If the child requires major school changes, such as special classrooms or therapies, peer relationships may be disrupted. In addition, children injured during this period may be aware of their deficits following the injury, which may affect their developing sense of self and competence.

The adolescent's reactions to the effects of the injury may be as significant a problem as the actual injury. Major social developments take place during adolescence and important educational decisions often made at this time may determine lifelong career patterns.

Summary

Developmental Effects

- The effects of a TBI must be interpreted in the context of the child's development
- Educators must be alert to the effects of a TBI on the child's subsequent development

Age and TBI Effects

- Children suffer greater effects of TBI than adults
- Younger children suffer greater effects than older children

4

Physical Effects of Traumatic Brain Injury

Neuropathology of TBI

An understanding of what happens to the brain in a traumatic injury helps us appreciate the long-term effects. At the time of injury, several forces act on the head to disrupt the integrity of the brain:

- *Impact*—When there is a blow to the skull or a sudden acceleration/deceleration action, such as when the head strikes the inside of a car, the brain continues to move within the skull. It slams against the inside of the skull at the point of impact and bounces back and forth so that the brain sustains blows on the opposite side as well. The impact at the site of the blow is referred to as a *coup*, and that which occurs at the opposite side of the head is the *contra-coup* injury.
- *Stretching*—Rotational forces acting within the brain at the time of impact stretch brain tissue. Such stretching affects the nerve fibers and the interconnecting network of nerve cells and fibers throughout the brain.

- *Abrasion*—The inside of the skull contains rough bony projections. When the brain moves back and forth inside the skull, it rubs against these rough spots, causing lacerated or torn tissue.

As a result of these forces, the brain is damaged in various ways. For example, an acceleration/deceleration event results in contusion, or bruising, of brain matter. The rotational forces stretch and tear fibers, many of which will be permanently damaged and some of which will die in the future. Damage from rotational forces is characterized by its diffuseness; that is, rather than being localized at the point of impact, it affects interconnecting fibers throughout the brain. Lacerations and the rotational forces not only damage brain matter, but disrupt the integrity of blood vessels, resulting in bleeding within the skull or brain.

The damage resulting from the above forces constitutes the *primary damage* occurring at the time of the accident as a direct result of the forces acting on the head. This is irreversible damage and will be the source of many of the long-term deficits. *Secondary damage* occurs as the brain reacts to the injury. This includes swelling of the brain from fluid buildup. Such swelling may disrupt blood flow as vessels are constricted, further straining nerve fibers and compressing brain tissue. As a result, further destruction of nerve cells may take place. Another source of secondary damage is *hemorrhage*, or bleeding, within the brain. A collection of blood can compress brain tissue, resulting in further damage. Finally, cells die when blood vessels that supply the brain are severed or constricted. In the early stages after the TBI, rapid improvement may be seen as secondary effects subside.

Characteristics of an Injured Brain

The long-term effects of TBI are more understandable if we consider the damage that has occurred. Damage is spread more widely within the brain than is generally realized. It is not unusual to hear a comment such as, "The left side of his brain was damaged because that's where he hit the steering wheel." In reality, the brain probably suffered from the impact at multiple sites of the surface (the coup and contra-coup effects). A blow to the head almost never injures a single site.

In children, the damage is diffuse, affecting multiple functions of the brain. It is important to realize that the diffuse damage from rotational forces occurs even in mild brain injuries with no loss of consciousness.

Damage to brain tissue is permanent, because brain tissue does not regenerate. The long-term neurological effects of the injury will be noted in tissue loss, atrophy of the *cortex* or outer layers of the brain, and possibly enlargement of the *ventricles* or spaces within the brain. These neurological characteristics of an injured brain have two major implications for the child's learning. First, many cognitive functions will be affected. Second, the influence of the TBI on the child's ability to learn will be long term, if not permanent.

Another characteristic of a brain that has been injured has implications for educators. As mentioned, a recently injured brain is susceptible to damage from subsequent trauma to the head. Because of this vulnerability, children with TBI must be protected from further injury, particularly in the first year after the initial injury. Generally, the student will be precluded from all contact sports or activities involving a risk for a blow to the head, such as water skiing or diving. A helmet for biking is imperative. Educators need to be sure of any applicable restrictions when the child returns to school.

Initial Effects of Injury: The Early Acute Phase

An injury to the brain may result in altered states of consciousness and memory disorders. Additionally, it may lead to medical, motor, and behavioral problems. Although these problems may resolve rather rapidly, it is important for educators to be familiar with them in order to understand the total recovery process.

Coma

Due to disruption of the brain stem functioning, the child is likely to be comatose following a TBI. Generally, the term *coma* is applied if the unconsciousness lasts for more than a short period (e.g., 1 hour). During a coma, the eyes are closed, no speech is evident, and no meaningful response to external stimuli can be evoked. This condition may last hours or weeks. A direct relationship has been established between the duration of the coma and the degree of later cognitive impairment. In addition to the duration, the degree of the coma is used to measure the severity of the TBI. The degree of coma may be quantified by using an observational scale, such as the *Glasgow Coma*

Scale (Teasdale & Jennette, 1974), which rates the patient's level of functioning in eye opening in response to stimuli, motor responsiveness to stimulation, and verbal responses (see Glossary). Another measure used to assess the child's state during the early period following a TBI is the *Rancho Los Amigos Scale* (Hagan, Malkmus, & Durham, 1979), which describes cognitive recovery using an 8-point scale (see Glossary). Both of these scales were originally developed with adults; modifications of these scales for children or other pediatric scales may be more widely used in the future (Yager, Johnston, & Seshia, 1990).

Posttraumatic Amnesia (PTA)

After emerging from a coma, the child may experience PTA. This term applies to an inability to store current events in totality. During the period of PTA, the child is unable to maintain a continuous memory for events that have happened during the day (e.g., the child may not remember what he or she had for breakfast or who came to visit that morning). PTA may last from a few to several days. Generally, PTA lasting a week or longer is associated with persistent cognitive impairments.

Medical Problems

In the early posttraumatic stage, the child may display a number of medical problems. Some occur as the result of injuries (e.g., broken bones, internal organ damage) sustained in the accident (especially in the case of motor vehicle accidents), whereas others develop due to the child's comatose condition. For example, children who are in a comatose condition may require *nasogastric* or *gastrostomy* tube feedings to ensure appropriate nutrient and fluid intake. Body temperature must be monitored for hypothermia (lowered temperature) or fever, which might indicate an infection. *Intracranial pressure* due to fluid buildup in the brain is monitored and treated since elevation may further damage brain tissue. Blood pressure is monitored and, if elevated, treated with *antihypertensive* medication (a drug that reduces blood pressure). Also, if the airways are obstructed, the child may be dependent on a tracheostomy tube to breathe.

Many of these medical problems are most pronounced in the first few weeks after the trauma. However, disorders related to thermal regulation and tracheostomy tube dependency may last for v months after the child has emerged from the coma.

Other Immediate Problems

Other immediate problems that are most pronounced in the early stages include severe motor problems, behavior abnormalities, and memory deficiencies. It is not uncommon for the child to exhibit only minimal voluntary movement immediately following the accident. Other motor problems during this period may include rigidity, tremors, *spasticity, ataxia* (loss of ability to coordinate smooth movements), or *apraxia* (inability to plan and carry out movements on command). The natural healing process combined with intensive physical and occupational therapies often resolve many of these motor problems rather rapidly.

In the early postcoma stage, the child is likely to exhibit several behavior abnormalities, such as extreme irritability, aggression, anxiety, or hypersensitivity to stimulation. As a result, the child may be difficult to work with because of resistance to therapies or daily caregiving routines. Uncontrolled or inappropriate emotions may also be present, or the child may lack any emotional expression. At this stage, signs of general confusion or disorientation are extremely common.

Severe memory disorders in the early postcoma stage include *retrograde amnesia,* in which the child is unable to recall events leading up to the accident. Commonly, children cannot recall the actual accident, and they may never regain the memory because the brain did not store these impressions. At this stage, they may also have difficulty remembering once-familiar persons or places.

Many of these early symptoms resolve rapidly, creating the impression that general recovery has taken place and that recovery will continue at the same, relatively rapid pace until the child is back to preinjury status. However, this early physical recovery is partly due to subsiding of the secondary trauma effects, whereas the primary tissue damage will persist and continue to affect future functioning. Families and friends should be aware that early rapid recovery is not an indication that long-term recovery will be rapid and complete. On the contrary, recovery from a TBI may never be complete. Therefore, recovery should be thought of as a continuum rather than an endpoint.

Persisting Effects of TBI

As mentioned, the first 6 months post-TBI is characterized by early rapid recovery, and many of the initial effects of the injury resolve so that the child may seem free of major aftereffects of the injury. However, 6 months to 1 year (or longer) after a moderate to severe TBI, the child may continue to exhibit a variety of medical, sensory, cognitive, and behavioral sequelae. These problems will be operating when the child returns to school and may persist for several years, if not for life. As a result, educators should be familiar with these problems so they can evaluate their implications and modify the student's educational program accordingly.

Physical Effects

A TBI may lead to problems related to endurance, comfort, regulation of physical functions, or impaired neurological status. For example, when returning to school, the student may have reduced stamina due to prolonged hospitalization and inactivity, seizures, or medications. Also, because of cognitive or motor deficits, routine activities may require extreme concentration, another cause of fatigue. Even if the child has made good physical recovery, the reduced stamina will prevent engaging in regular preaccident routines. Reduced stamina can continue to be a problem for a year or more, preventing the student from returning to school full time.

After a TBI, a child is also more likely to develop seizures than noninjured children. Approximately 5% of children who have suffered a serious TBI develop seizures (Hauser, 1983). These seizures, sometimes referred to as *posttraumatic epilepsy*, can usually be controlled by medication. Even if the child has not had any seizures, the neurologist may prescribe medication for up to a year following the injury to reduce the possibility of seizures developing. Parents should rely on the physician's advice as to when the child can be taken off the medication. Side effects such as drowsiness and impaired cognition should be discussed with the physician.

Headaches also commonly occur following a TBI. The child's physician may treat such headaches with mild analgesics or prescribe rest periods. Parents and teachers should rely on the advice of the physician for the treatment of headaches, and should report any increase in severity or frequency. In addition, they should watch for signs of headaches in children who are not old enough to report their occurrence.

PHYSICAL EFFECTS 19

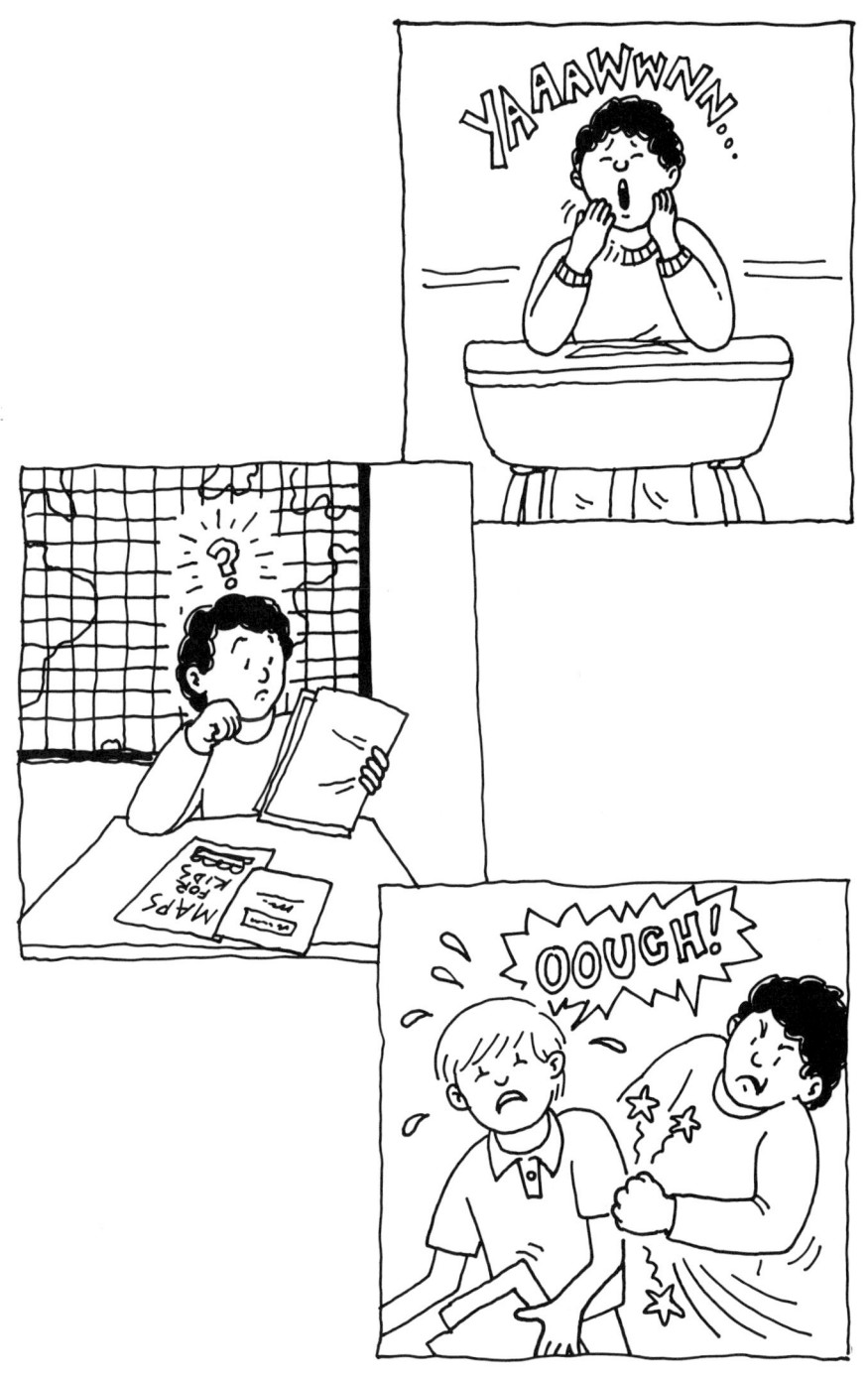

Brain centers that control appetite, temperature, and certain types of hormone production may be damaged and cause the child to experience some of the following difficulties. These uncommon, but very significant, difficulties include growth problems because of disruption in growth hormone production; eating disorders because of deficiencies of appetite control; development of diabetes; and serious temperature shifts due to problems with the body's thermostat. Persisting problems involving the muscular system may result in skeletal deformities, requiring careful monitoring by an orthopedic specialist.

Sensory Effects

Common sensory problems after a TBI include hearing and vision deficits. Frequently, the ear is damaged during a TBI. In cases of damage to the middle ear, a conductive hearing loss may result, whereas damage to the inner ear or the auditory pathways may lead to a sensorineural hearing loss. Although the conductive hearing loss may resolve itself over time, the sensorineural hearing loss may show some but never complete recovery. Because of the prevalence of hearing loss after a TBI, children should undergo complete audiological evaluations.

Over half of the children injured experience vision problems, including blurred or double vision and visual field defects. Whereas the first two often improve over the first 6 months, field defects may persist. If so, the child will experience a restricted field of vision either to the side or above or below the glance. It is important that any child who has suffered a TBI receive a comprehensive ophthalmologic examination.

Cognitive Effects

Children with TBI typically demonstrate long-term cognitive problems. These are particularly significant because they affect the child's daily functioning and have a major impact on educational achievement. Long-term cognitive sequelae may include memory and attention impairments, intellectual deficits, and language problems, as well as higher level problem-solving deficits.

The most common and long lasting of these cognitive deficits is memory impairment. This is particularly serious for a child because memory problems affect educational progress. Thus, if long-term storage and retrieval are adversely affected, the child may not be able to remember material that was learned prior to the accident. Although the child may eventually relearn old material, severe short-term memory problems will significantly interfere with new learning.

Memory problems will also significantly affect the child's noninstructional school activities and daily functioning. For example, during the schoolday, memory problems may cause the child to have difficulty recalling the day's schedule, homework assignments, or the appropriate materials to bring to class. Furthermore, because daily living activities may no longer be automatic, the child may experience difficulties at home with usual routines such as dressing, preparing meals, or completing chores.

In addition to memory, intellectual functions are often affected by a TBI, generally in proportion to the severity of the injury. Although it is not uncommon for children with mild to moderate injuries eventually to return to preinjury IQ levels, children with severe injuries may show only partial recovery of previous skills. However, educators should be cautioned that, despite recovery of measured IQ, children with TBI may continue to have problems with new learning due to deficits in problem solving, reasoning, and memory that are not reflected in IQ scores.

Children who have sustained even a mild TBI may have difficulties with attention and concentration. If unable to attend to or concentrate on the task at hand, the child's ability to function in school and learn new material is affected. Furthermore, children who had difficulty in this area prior to their accidents will encounter more difficulty after their TBI.

Language Effects

Whereas obvious communication problems (e.g., severe motor-speech problems and lack of speech) that were present in the early postcoma period may resolve within a few weeks, the child may experience long-term problems in expressive language and comprehension. For example, following a TBI, children commonly have difficulty with word retrieval, leading to their talking around a subject or using indefinite words. Also, difficulty retrieving strings of words may lead to verbal fluency problems in demand situations, causing children problems with the pragmatic aspects of language or the way they use language in conversation. For example, they may be unable to take turns in conversation, be concise, or keep a conversation going. Residual motor-speech problems may result in a slow rate of speech or in *dysarthria,* which is characterized by imprecise articulation that reduces intelligibility, harsh voice quality, and greater nasality or breathiness. Furthermore, language comprehension, which may superficially appear intact, can break down in complex listening situations (e.g., when the instructional material is unfamiliar, when verbal directions are complex or given rapidly, or when involved in group conversations).

It is important to recognize that the less obvious language deficits are not fully revealed in a one-to-one testing situation under ideal conditions. Such an examination also does not necessarily demonstrate the child's ability to acquire new vocabulary or language concepts. All these problems may not show up until the child experiences difficulty learning new language skills at an age-expected rate.

Difficulty comprehending complex language and academic material will interfere with the child's ability to be successful in school. In addition to language deficits, underlying cognitive deficits in attention, concentration, and memory will affect how the child functions in less structured situations, such as group verbal interchanges. The child may have difficulty communicating with peers because of disorganized or socially inappropriate verbal behavior. These difficulties in social situations will spill over into the child's self-esteem and overall psychosocial functioning.

Behavioral/Emotional Effects

Teachers should be aware that a number of behavioral and emotional problems may occur as a result of a TBI. Several years after an injury, over 50% of children suffering severe TBI demonstrate behavioral problems that emerged after the injury, and as many as a third of those with mild TBI demonstrate new behavioral problems (Brown, Chadwick, Shaffer, Rutter, & Traub, 1981). Some of these problems are directly related to the injury; TBI alters the way in which the brain reacts and regulates responses. For example, damage, particularly to the vulnerable frontal lobes, leads to deficits in the important executive cognitive abilities, such as planning, organization, and problem solving. These cognitive impairments may be noted in overt behaviors such as disinhibition and problems with planning. Other behaviors may represent the child's reactions to the injury and resulting deficits. Included here are problems stemming from lengthy hospitalization. However, even the way in which the child expresses these reactive problems may be moderated by the impaired brain. Other behavioral problems are those that were present before, but are now magnified by the TBI. Thus, behaviors that were previously only annoying may become problematic.

Behavioral disturbances commonly include overactivity and impulsivity. Young children may act quite aggressively and, due to disinhibition, say or do things that are socially inappropriate. Furthermore, the child may lack self-direction, being unable to start or stop an activity without assistance, behaviors that teachers may erroneously interpret as lack of motivation. Problems of fleeting concentration make it difficult for the child to attend to an activity or instructions. Other problems may include apathy or increased helplessness, which can make the child very demanding.

Another problem, arising directly from the injury to the brain, is characterized by an inability on the part of injured children to recognize that they have suffered any impairments from the injury. This neurologically based denial of injury effects is *not* a psychological defense, but represents a true inability to recognize the physical, cognitive, or behavioral impairments that are obvious to others. This inability to realize the deficits makes it difficult for children to understand how their behavior is troublesome to others, and to recognize that they are different from before or are behaving differently from the norm. For example, the child may be unable to recognize that behaviors such as acting out sexually, threatening other students, or swearing are inappropriate, and cannot understand why school personnel want to limit the child's contact with other students.

Behavioral management is vital for dealing with behavioral problems, even when these are related to abnormal brain functioning, since the child's ability to function in school and community will be hindered by behavioral problems. (Specific programming suggestions for dealing with behavioral problems in school are discussed in Chapter 9 of this guide.)

The treatment of behavioral problems associated with TBI often needs to be multifaceted. In some cases, medication is useful, but it must be handled carefully, taking into account the child's neurological problems, anticipated side effects, and other medication prescribed. Ideally, the medication should be monitored by a physician knowledgeable about TBI. In addition, counseling is particularly important for adolescents who might have to make changes in career goals.

Academic Effects

Although the academic effects of a TBI vary from child to child, some problems are widespread. For example, mathematics skills are sensitive to TBI effects and may be severely impaired immediately after the injury. Computational skills may be regained relatively quickly, but deficits in mathematical reasoning and problem solving may persist. Similarly, reading ability may be impaired immediately after a TBI. Decoding abilities may appear to recover fairly soon, but long-term deficits in reading comprehension are common, particularly among children injured at a young age, and those who have sustained severe injuries. The deficits in higher level cognitive skills, memory, and mental processing, contribute to these academic problems.

Teachers should be cautioned that, even though the child scores at grade level on achievement tests, this may not accurately reflect actual functioning. Individual achievement tests are not good indicators of a child's ability to learn in the classroom following a TBI because these tests are given under ideal conditions and, therefore, do not reflect the kinds of difficulty a child may face in a busy classroom with less guidance and structure. Also, achievement measures may reflect overlearned skills that show little impairment following injury. Thus, it is only when the child fails to make appropriate academic gains that the problems are recognized.

Academic functioning deficits coupled with long-term behavioral and cognitive problems prevent many children from continuing in a regular or unmodified classroom. Before the legislated expansion of special education services, students with TBI required modifications in their educational program. Many were either retained, or received remedial or special services, or dropped out of school (Klonoff, Low, & Clark, 1977). Recent evidence on the academic effects of TBI further support this notion. In spite of adequate performance on individual achievements tests, the majority of students who have sustained moderate to severe injuries are served within modified regular classes. For example, 2 years after their injury, only one-fourth of the children who had a TBI that resulted in impaired consciousness for longer than 24 hours were able to function in a regular class (Ewing-Cobbs, Iovino, Fletcher, Miner, & Levin, 1991). In the population of students we work with, over half of those who suffer moderate to severe TBI receive special education services, including placement in classrooms for students with learning disabilities, mental retardation, or physical impairments, or the provision of learning disabilities resource services or consultative services from specialists in behavior disorders (Mira, 1989).

Interaction of Problems Resulting from TBI

The cognitive, motor, and behavioral problems resulting from a TBI interact to create more significant long-term difficulties. For example, problems related to carrying out motor operations quickly or efficiently interact with cognitive deficits or attention and memory in the classroom. Specifically, the inability to quickly copy all assignments from the board may mean that the student goes home without knowing what homework needs to be completed that evening. Similarly, reduced speed in completing a task may cause the student to forget what the entire task is before being able to finish it. For these reasons, the child is allowed fewer opportunities to respond in the classroom, where the emphasis is on performance.

Motor problems also affect social interactions with peers. Having to be let out from one class early to get to the next on time, precludes the student from the informal between-class interchanges with peers. Also, peers may view incoordination and dysarthric speech as distasteful.

When unable to perform successfully in an unmodified classroom, the student with TBI may react inappropriately because of judgment difficulties and disinhibition. Furthermore, such children may not be able to articulate to the teacher that they are experiencing distress because the instructions were too complex or presented too quickly. Instead, they are prone to act out, produce poor work, or eventually withdraw from the task.

Other examples of the interaction of problems are seen in the way in which language difficulties affect academic functioning or interpersonal relationships. For example, difficulty with word retrieval or verbal and written formulation may impair the child's ability to express what has been learned in the classroom. These same problems can limit the child's ability to interact with peers. Thus, educators need to view the way in which the child will function as a result of several deficits working together rather than fragmented isolated deficits.

Summary

Mechanism of Injury

- Primary damage
  - Acceleration/deceleration on impact, leading to contusion
  - Rotational forces, which stretch nerve fibers
  - Abrasion that lacerates brain tissue

- Secondary damage
  - Swelling
  - Hemorrhage
  - Disruption of blood flow

Characteristics of Damage

- Diffuse rather than focal
- Multiple sites and multiple functions affected
- Permanent

Initial Effects of Injury

- Coma
- Posttraumatic amnesia
- Medical problems
- Motor problems

Persisting Effects of TBI

- Physical
- Sensory
- Cognitive
- Language
- Behavioral/emotional
- Academic

5

Psychosocial Effects of Traumatic Brain Injury

Types of Psychosocial Problems

Psychosocial difficulties are the most significant of the TBI effects for children and adolescents. Unfortunately, these problems persist. They are not easily treated because they not only are related to the actual injury, but are compounded by subsequent problems with social relationships and success in school. Psychosocial difficulties cluster in several areas, described below.

Disorders in Family Relationships

A child's severe illness and subsequent lengthy rehabilitation may alter family roles. For example, greater need for supervision or restrictions on activity set the injured child apart from siblings. Brothers and sisters may resent the excessive parental attention the injured child receives. If the injured child is the survivor of an accident in which other family members were killed, consequent difficulties in relationships among remaining members may ensue.

Peer Relationships

Following a moderate to severe TBI, children and adolescents experience significant disruptions in their friendships. Sometimes the peer group reconstitutes without the injured child. Also, upon return to school, the child's resocialization may be difficult because of activity limitations imposed by the disabilities.

Friends who rallied at the time of injury may drift away if the child's behavior or cognitive deficits impair effective functioning in groups. For example, problems of memory, concentration, and cognition lead to behaviors that peers view negatively. The injured child may no longer be able to interact in the quick-witted way that adolescents, in particular, admire. The child may be overwhelmed by social interactions requiring rapid processing of complex stimuli and may withdraw from social activities.

Problems of Independence

TBI can dramatically alter the child's or adolescent's ability to function as independently as before. Greater dependency may be a residual of the constant caregiving required after the injury, or may reflect restrictions from physical limitations or impaired judgment. The child's failure to recognize deficit-imposed limitations may cause the child to view parents as unreasonably restrictive, thereby bringing about serious family conflicts.

Affective Disturbances

Changes in the way emotional reactions are experienced and expressed are common following a TBI. Irritability and depression are common upon recognizing the loss of one's former abilities. After several years of unsatisfactory peer relationships, limited achievement, and the failure of others to recognize the cognitive deficits that are hindering functioning, students may become so distressed that they contemplate suicide. This risk is so great that teachers must view any talk or action hinting at suicide as a serious reaction by the student.

Realizing Career Goals

Physical or cognitive residuals may mean changes in college or job goals. An anticipated athletic scholarship may be put out of reach, or college plans may have to be altered. These issues are particularly significant for students who are injured in the later school years.

Age Considerations

The ways in which long-term psychosocial problems develop vary with the child's age. Among younger children, psychosocial problems may not emerge for several years as it takes parents and teachers a long time to recognize that the child is merely relying on previous skills. In the meantime, the child is expected to behave as before the accident. Even if vaguely aware of not measuring up to these unaltered expectations, the child may be unable to change the situation. The result may be erosion of the child's self-esteem, or reduced classroom effort.

For adolescents who have sustained a TBI, the subsequent psychosocial difficulties are often more debilitating than the actual effects of the injury. The ability of the family, school, and student to realize the effects of the TBI and to deal with them realistically is particularly critical in this age group. Indeed, the psychosocial problems of TBI for adolescents are so complex that they warrant separate consideration.

Issues in Adolescent TBI

Many variables interact to create long-standing and serious psychosocial problems for adolescents who sustain a TBI. A major factor is the inability of many families and educators to recognize and deal openly and realistically with the residual deficits of TBI in adolescents. When students are unable to recognize the deficits, because of the organic denial mentioned in Chapter 4, they do not see the need for remediation or behavior changes, and are therefore hampered in developing a realistic picture of their new self. On the other hand, if adolescents are aware of their difficulty with new learning, while teachers act as if no problems exist, the students must face their problems alone.

Following a TBI, adolescents have to deal with the same issues of peer relations, sexuality, independence, and life goals as their peers. However, cognitive deficits may diminish their abilities to problem solve effectively in these areas. In most instances, the issue of adolescent sexuality is openly ignored following a TBI, yet this is the period of maximal sexual interest, learning, and activity. Following a TBI, the adolescent may be cut off from peers, who are the major source of information about sexual matters. Physical deficits or reduced stamina will interfere with sexual function. Problems of impaired judgment and impulsiveness have grave consequences for sexual behavior. For example, these problems may lead to uncritical choice of partners, inappropriate selection of time or place, or disregard for contraception.

Families may respond to the adolescent's judgment deficits by increasing restrictions on activities. Parents may impose curfews, or insist that a brother or sister accompany the adolescent at all times. Adolescents do not welcome increased supervision, or restrictions on their movement around the community. Thus, increased restraints become a source of conflict within the family and may eventually cause the adolescent to become depressed.

Under these circumstances, families may unwittingly contribute to the adolescent's psychosocial difficulties by overprotection. Parents' difficulty letting go may continue even after the student leaves high school and moves away to attend college or live independently. It is not unusual to find parents, even of these older students, answering questions for them in the clinic or reminding them to hang up their coats.

Within a few months after the injury, the adolescent may look unchanged superficially, showing no overt deficits that might otherwise alert parents and teachers to the difficulties the student is experiencing. Indeed, behaviors such as argumentativeness, irritability, and poor judgment arising from the injury may be viewed as typical adolescent behavior. Also, academic problems may be misinterpreted as motivation deficits. In many instances, parents receive inadequate help from professionals after the injury in learning how to distinguish behavioral problems related to the injury from developmental characteristics of a given age.

Teachers also have difficulty understanding what part of the behavior is related to the TBI and what is adolescent behavior. Thus, it is not uncommon during a meeting with a parent about the student's postinjury needs for a teacher to dismiss certain behaviors by saying, "He was just like this before the injury." The implication of this comment is that (a) since the behavior is not a direct part of the TBI, special programming to deal with it is not required, or (b) the behavior is the fault of the student or the family.

Another source of difficulty, especially for high school students, arises when adults do not understand adolescents' diminished capacity to make sound decisions or respond accurately to their own behavior. At this level, teachers assign a great deal of responsibility to students for making decisions about their own educational programs. Following a TBI, many adolescents are unable to meet these expectations and cannot recognize when their behavior is out of line or predict its consequences.

Following a TBI, their judgment defects and organically based denial of problems may preclude adolescents from effectively determining schedules, level of classes in which to enroll, and even amount of stamina. Therefore, adolescents may require that behavioral expectations and rules be spelled out in as much detail as is typical for younger students. The issue of independent decision making is another area in which educators and families receive little preparation or assistance.

An issue seldom addressed with post-TBI adolescents is substance abuse, although alcohol use and abuse are strongly implicated as causes of TBI. Blood alcohol levels are seldom checked in adolescents at the time of trauma. However, about half of injured adolescents have been found to demonstrate blood alcohol levels above the legal level for intoxication (Kraus & Nourjah, 1989). Presence of alcohol in the blood at the time of the trauma complicates recovery and intensifies neurological and cognitive sequelae.

For many reasons, adolescents may return to alcohol or other drugs after a TBI. For example, they may try to mask the hurt of alienation of friends, family conflicts, and the loss of skills. Alcohol and other post-TBI drug use can be particularly disastrous. Even occasional use of recreational drugs post-TBI is dangerous. Most drugs inhibit recovery and interact with the residual deficits in ways the student does not anticipate, making the risk of a second TBI high. For example, seizure thresholds are altered and cognitive and motor problems and judgment defects are intensified.

The School's Role in Psychosocial Outcome

Within the school, we can do much to help the students' long-range adjustment. Primarily, it is important that we not take recovery for granted even though the student appears normal. When complicating motor or cognitive deficits are not recognized in the classroom, the student may exhibit behavioral outbursts. For example, if a student with reduced mental processing speed is not given enough time to complete an assignment and is penalized for the deficit, an emotional outburst may be understandable. As we have emphasized, sub-

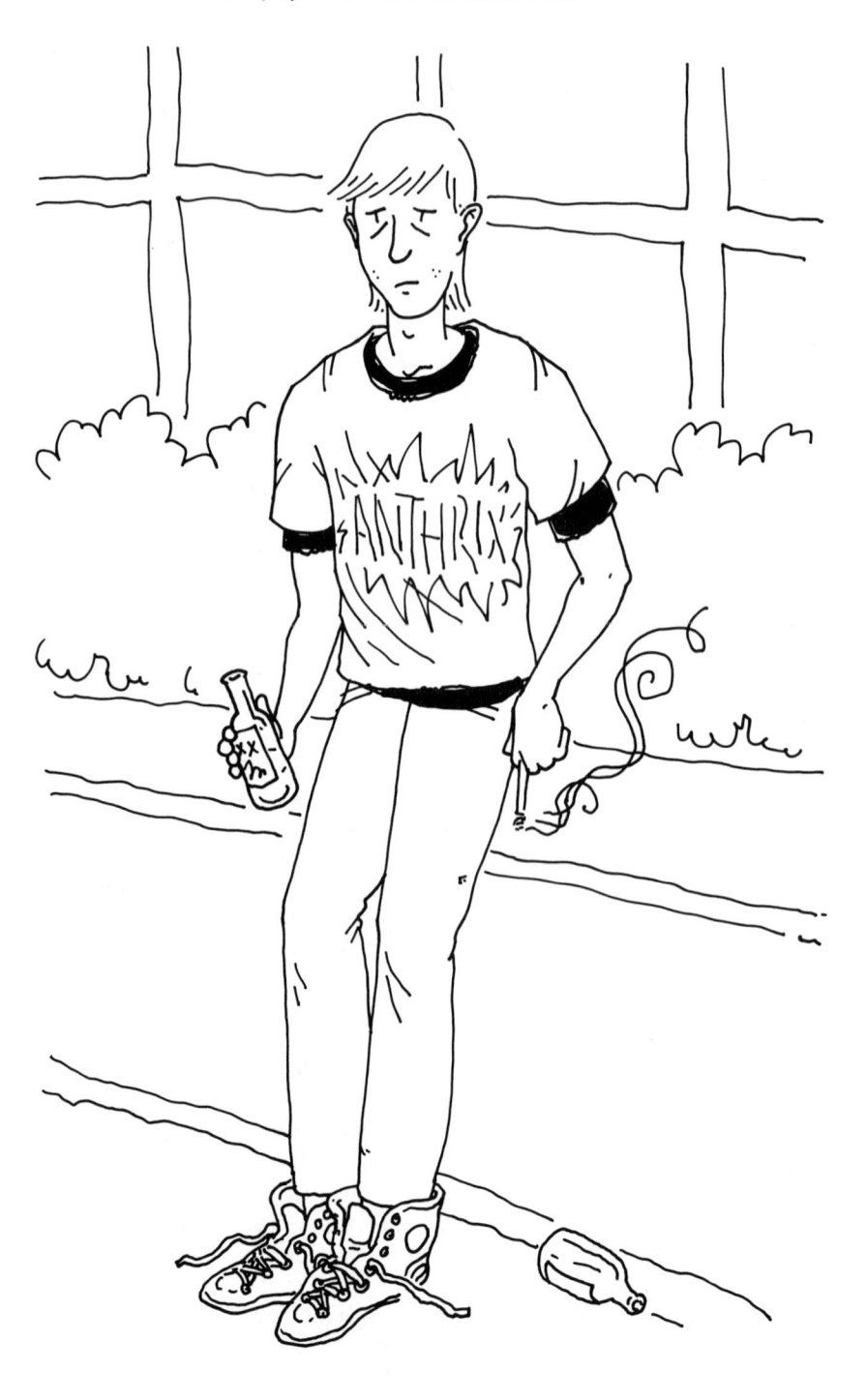

tle cognitive deficits often interfere with effective classroom behavior. It is important not to misinterpret behaviors, for example, not to misinterpret problems with self-initiation as motivational deficits.

While recognizing that many of the behavioral problems exhibited by a student with TBI stem from the functioning of a damaged brain, environmental events that can trigger behavioral outbursts may be considered. Examples include excessive stimulation, changes from expected routines, unpredicted events, too many instructions, or lack of clear expectations. Educators can help the student function better by altering the environment or exploring new ways for the student to react to these events. Ongoing counseling at school is important for students with TBI as a way to anticipate problems rather than waiting for adjustment problems to erupt.

Educators can make a major contribution to a student's adjustment and recovery by accurately identifying deficits and openly articulating their presence and impact, both with families and with the student. Thus, educators must offer clear feedback about the accuracy of work and appropriateness of behavior, and implement programming accordingly.

Summary

Areas of Psychosocial Difficulties

- Family relationships
- Peer relationships
- Independent functioning
- Career goals
- Emotional state

Issues for Adolescents

- Recognition of deficits
- Meeting adolescent problems with diminished problem-solving ability
- Activity restrictions

- Overprotection
- Distinguishing post-TBI effects from normal adolescent behavior
- Inability to make sound decisions
- Drugs and alcohol
- Sexuality

6

Continuum of Treatment for Traumatic Brain Injury

Components of a Comprehensive Program

Acute Care Phase

Treatment of a head injury usually begins at the injury scene and continues in the emergency room of a local hospital or a regional trauma center. Such a center offers 24-hour emergency teams and state-of-the-art technology. The disadvantage is that families often have to travel considerable distances to be with their injured child. This adds additional stress to the shock of having a child seriously injured.

The child usually remains in the intensive care unit (ICU) while comatose or until medical problems requiring 24-hour monitoring are resolved. When neurologically stable and emerging from the coma, the child is transferred from the ICU to an acute care rehabilitation unit of the hospital.

Postacute Care

Postacute care begins in a rehabilitation unit, which provides a comprehensive array of services and therapies designed to restore the injured person's functional potential. Typically, patients receive physical, occupational, and speech therapies.

The child will be measured for splints, braces, or a wheelchair, if necessary. The need for augmentative communication is also assessed, if the child is unable to speak. In addition, posttraumatic amnesia is monitored, and all caregivers attempt to get or keep the patient oriented to time and place.

The postacute care period can vary from a few days to months, depending on progress. Some hospitals discharge patients who are medically stable but have reached a progress plateau. This is done to conserve insurance benefits for the time when the child has progressed enough to benefit from therapies again.

Outpatient Rehabilitation

Acute care inpatient rehabilitation may be followed by a period of outpatient rehabilitation involving return visits to a rehabilitation hospital at regular intervals (sometimes daily) to continue required therapies. At this point, the child may need only speech therapy or occupational therapy. If outpatient therapy is undertaken at a hospital located closer to the patient's home, communication takes place between therapists at the former and the new center via transmission of records and direct conferences.

Residential rehabilitation programs have become more widely available in the past 5 years, and may be the best alternative for some children. While offering the advantage of comprehensive and intense treatment designed and implemented by a highly skilled team of professionals, the expense and further separation and dislocation of families must be seriously considered.

School Reentry

If long-term residential placement is not necessary, students with TBI will probably resume their education. At first, homebound teaching may be provided while the student receives outpatient therapy at the rehabilitation facility. Homebound education sessions are short and flexible so that outpatient therapy and education can proceed simultaneously. Instruction may also be tailored to accommodate the reduced stamina that is typical for students with TBI.

CONTINUUM OF TREATMENT 37

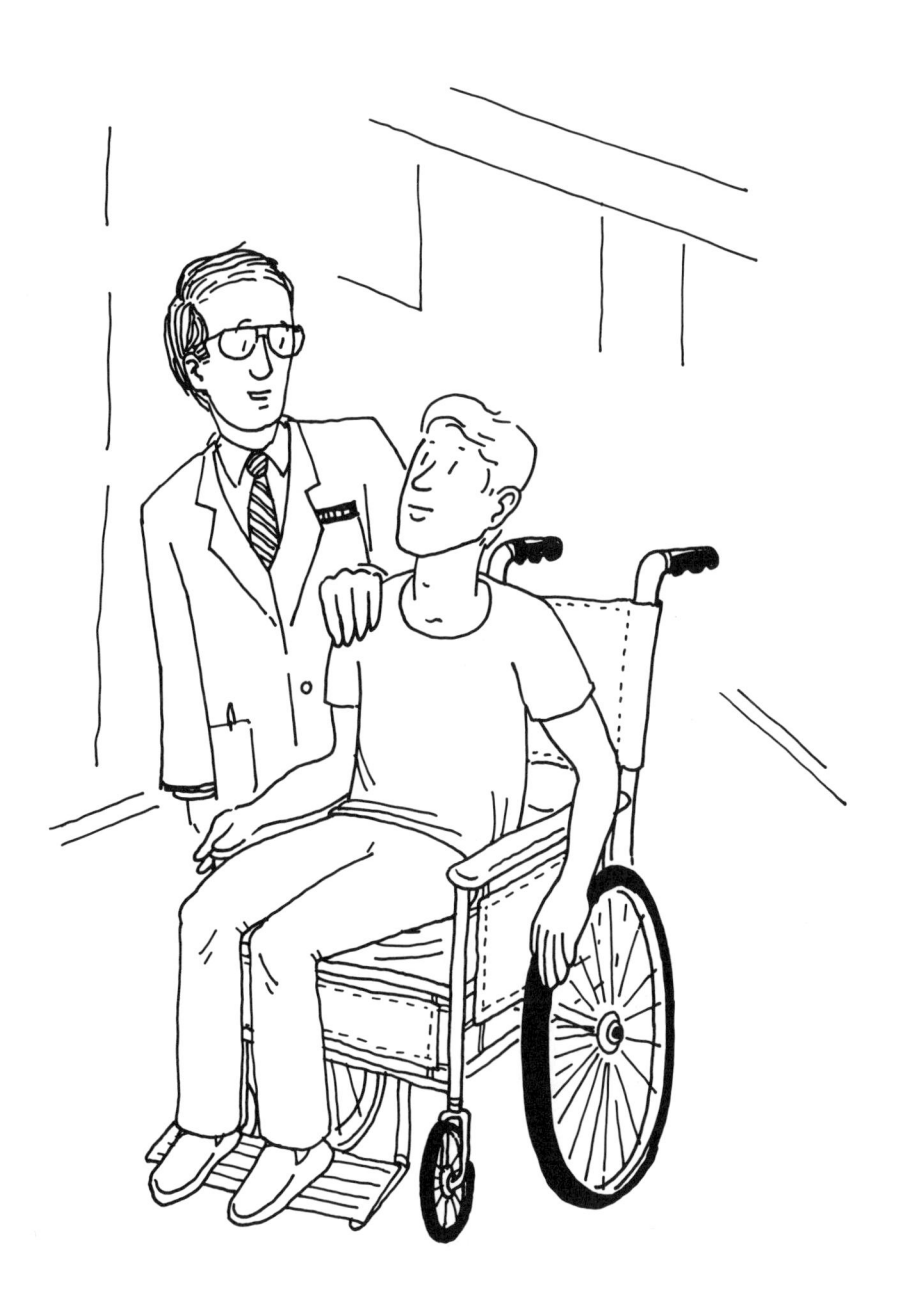

School reentry can be affected by many variables, some child centered, others more administrative. For example, sometimes reentry is dictated by the school calendar rather than the child's readiness. A child who is ready to return to school in mid-May, for example, is facing a school year that is winding down. Thus, end-of-the-year field trips and other activities that culminate each school year may not lend themselves to the solid learning appropriate for the child in this phase. Instead, homebound teaching sessions may be lengthened or summer school planned. In some cases, parental eagerness for the child to get on with life may be a significant factor in premature school reentry.

Ideally, the child's needs are the highest priority in setting the time for school reentry. If educators use the specified criteria for reentry, school calendars and parental eagerness may be deferred in favor of child readiness.

To benefit from school placement, students with TBI should be able to do the following (Cohen, Joyce, Rhoades, & Welks, 1985, pp. 384–385):

1. Attend to a task for 10–15 minutes
2. Tolerate 20–30 minutes of general classroom stimulation (movement, distractions, noises)
3. Function within a group of two or more students
4. Engage in some type of meaningful communication
5. Follow simple (one- or two-step) directions
6. Give evidence of learning potential

After this readiness assessment, a review of medical records, follow-ups, and summaries of rehabilitation therapies is a logical starting point for beginning an initial plan. The child's needs in the school environment and curriculum may be accommodated in a variety of ways. Sometimes the homebound teacher continues to teach the child, but the sessions are conducted at school rather than at home.

How Schools Can Interact with Hospitals

During the acute care phase following TBI, teachers and students will probably send cards, letters, pictures, and maybe audiotapes or videotapes to the hospital. Hospital personnel usually display these communications in their efforts to help the child remember things prior to the accident. Posttraumatic amnesia is common, and communication from home and school are powerful tools for combatting its effects.

Significant people from school may be able to schedule short, regular visits to the rehabilitation unit. For example, teachers and the school principal or counselor may call or visit to keep abreast of the student's recovery rate and to begin setting the stage at school for eventual reentry. This is also a time to be sure that parents have given informed consent to exchange records between school and hospital.

Hospital personnel may ask for school records to determine preinjury levels of performance and behavior, instead of asking parents. Although parental report is usually fairly accurate, it is nonetheless beneficial to verify and amplify it by reviewing copies of school achievement test data, attendance records, and anecdotal information that may provide keys to more effective rehabilitation.

As postacute rehabilitation continues, the involvement of school personnel gradually intensifies. Questions regarding when to prepare for reentry and what modifications will be needed in both the school environment and the student's schedule and curriculum are best answered by being familiar with hospital rehabilitation progress.

At this point, a designated *school case coordinator* or manager can become active. Increasing the school's visibility at the hospital usually results in getting needed information for school planning purposes. Attendance at treatment planning and review meetings is one way to secure information. In addition, participation in discharge planning meetings is nearly essential.

If long-term residential treatment is the most appropriate option for the student at the end of acute care rehabilitation, school professionals should make an effort to stay informed about progress there. The residential programs that have proliferated during the last few years often have their own school systems, run by on-site certified teachers and other educational personnel. Sometimes, these programs are so extensive that teachers from the local school system are based there full time. Ideally, such programs work with the nearest local school system to phase their residents in and begin school reentry as a part of the total residential treatment plan. If a student is placed in such a program, someone from the student's home school district must be in touch with teachers at the residential facility. Often it is necessary for the home school to initiate communication to guarantee an efficient "feedback loop."

Issues in Financing the Rehabilitation/ Recovery Program

There are major questions regarding the financing of a program that provides the necessary services for a student with TBI. The expense of an appropriate, comprehensive program can deplete a district's special education budget. The issue is clouded because there is no clear demarcation between rehabilitation services and services that are a necessary part of the child's education.

Many school systems regard school reentry as the starting point for assuming financial responsibility for needed therapies. Therefore, therapies that occur on an outpatient basis (before school reentry) are considered by the school district as rehabilitation and, thus, the responsibility of the parents or the insurance company. Even if a child is receiving homebound instruction during this period, a school may not assume financial responsibility for therapies until the child has recovered sufficiently for reentry. These assumptions about the school's responsibility may be challenged, however, as the new mandate is implemented.

It is erroneous to believe that the family's insurance will cover therapies if these are not provided by the school. Many insurance programs have a lifetime limit. The cost of inpatient care may have consumed these benefits at alarming rates.

In cases where the student attends school in a residential treatment setting, the child's home school district may pay for the educational segment of treatment. Such arrangements are usually handled on a case-by-case basis. Questions arise when the home school system can provide the needed services but the parents opt for a residential placement:

- Is the school system still responsible for paying educational costs?
- Can the school system withhold payment for services provided outside the district when the same level and quality of service could be provided in the home school setting?
- Where and when does rehabilitation end and education begin?
- Are the two inextricable for TBI students?

The high cost of educating and rehabilitating students with TBI will force school districts to answer these and other questions about where school responsibility begins and ends, especially in severe, long-term cases. Because there are no guidelines, schools vary widely in the types and extent of services they provide. These issues relating to financial responsibility for the many services required need to be resolved as districts implement the new mandate.

Summary

Stages of Treatment

- Acute care
- Postacute care
- Outpatient rehabilitation
- School reentry

Criteria for School Reentry

- Attend to task for 10–15 minutes
- Tolerate 20–30 minutes of classroom stimulation
- Function in a group of two or more
- Engage in meaningful communication
- Follow simple directions
- Give evidence of learning potential

7

Planning for School Reentry

Framework for Developing an Educational Plan Following a TBI

Traumatic brain injury is now identified as a separate disability category within special education (PL 101-476). Although we do not know how this new special education provision will be translated into programs by individual states, we do know that special education administrators, teachers, and diagnostic staff will need further information and training about TBI. In addition, school districts will need to establish plans for delivery of services to these children. An important element in providing services to children with TBI is the reentry planning that must take place prior to the child's return to school, beginning while the child is in the hospital.

Establishing Communication Between Rehabilitation Professionals and Schools

It is essential to establish communication between educators and rehabilitation staff as soon as the child is medically stable. School personnel should take the initiative to talk to the child's doctors and therapists, hospital social worker, hospital teacher, psychologist, and neuropsychologist to gain information about the child and to start planning for the child's return to school.

As mentioned in Chapter 6, it is helpful for school staff to observe the child during therapy or in the hospital school to gain a better understanding of how the child is functioning. Such visits also offer an opportunity to establish communication links with therapists and medical staff.

A predischarge planning meeting is usually arranged by the hospital before the child goes home to review the child's functioning and needs in all areas and to make recommendations for continued therapy. If possible, parents and school diagnostic and teaching staff should attend this meeting. In addition to receiving information, school staff can provide information about what resources will be available in the child's school and community. In some cases, this conference can serve as the school's prediagnostic staff meeting.

When the child is discharged from the hospital, school personnel should obtain the following information about the child:

- Complete medical history
- Present medical status
- Current fine- and gross-motor functioning
- Current neurologic status
- Results of an in-hospital neuropsychological exam
- Summary of the child's present communication/language skills
- Complete report of the child's current cognitive functioning

(See also Appendix B for a physical facilities and planning checklist that school personnel should fill out prior to the child's return to school.)

Appropriate Educational Goals for Students with TBI

Realistic goals are critical to planning an effective educational program. It is unrealistic, for example, to expect the educational program to return all children to preinjury status or better. It is also unrealistic to assume that all children can return to school and pick up at pre-injury levels. A more realistic goal is to develop a specialized program that will maximize learning, facilitate the return of as much functioning as possible, and allow for continuing progress.

Critical Elements that Should Be in Place in Schools

Several elements should be in place before the child reenters the school system. These include the following:

1. *Provision for the child's safety.* Impulsiveness and poor judgment may place the child in dangerous situations. In addition, coordination and balance deficits, along with cognitive deficits, enhance the child's risk for sustaining another injury. Therefore, the child requires increased supervision, modification of the physical environment, and reduced access to harmful agents (e.g., fumes from paint and solvents, chemicals, and nonprescriptive drugs and alcohol) to which he or she is now more susceptible because of the altered nature of the impaired brain.

2. *A staff that is well informed.* School personnel should be informed not only about the returning child, but about the effects of TBI in general.

3. *Staff and facilities to provide a program of the necessary intensity.* The program needs to take into account the child's cognitive deficits and needs for language and motor therapies that will enhance learning in the classroom.

4. *An environment that is sufficiently controlled.* A controlled environment allows the student to receive instruction with as much one-to-one direction as needed, while interfering or competing stimuli are reduced as needed.

5. *Provision of special equipment.* Needed augmentative communication, response enhancement, and locomotion equipment must be in place before the child returns to school.

6. *Ability to design and implement a behavioral management program to deal with interfering behavioral deficits.* School personnel must be committed to securing these services consultatively if they are not available within the school.

7. *Knowledge of the TBI resources that are available to schools.* School staff should be aware of state-level special education consultants, state and national head injury associations, and regional specialists in TBI.

8. *Planned provisions for frequent communication among staff.* Planned interchange allows for the generation of new ideas, provides mutual support, and aids in identifying those parts of the program that are not working as planned.

Barriers that Can Impede Successful School Reintegration

Several barriers can impede the successful school reintegration of children with TBI. These factors are reviewed here to help school staff recognize them if present in their own school and to plan accordingly.

1. *Lack of staff training.* One of the main barriers to successfully reintegrating the student with a TBI is that school staff generally lack training in the area of TBI and, thus, do not fully understand the needs of children with TBI. Such a lack of knowledge is due to the fact that the professional preparation of educators and psychologists does not generally address TBI. Thus, school staff must take it upon themselves to obtain the needed training and information about TBI.

2. *Addition of new staff without training.* Even if the school staff is trained prior to the child's reentry, it is equally important that any newly hired staff, including those who will serve as substitute teachers in the child's classroom, receive training about TBI. Therefore, a mechanism should be in place to ensure that new staff are informed about the specific needs of the child with TBI. This may include making a designated person responsible for ensuring that any new staff member receive needed training.

3. *Lack of flexibility in program planning.* Rigid adherence to school calendars, schedules, categories of handicapping conditions, or computer-generated Individualized Educational Plans (IEPs), make it virtually impossible to provide appropriate programming for each student with a TBI. Therefore, the school staff must work with the school district's administrators to establish a program that meets the student's needs. This may include providing summer instruction, arranging the schedule to meet the student's needs, offering special education services appropriate for the handicapping condition, and foregoing computer-generated IEPs in favor of a hand-written IEP if the needed goals are not found in the computer program. Overall, if the staff first identifies the specific needs of the child and then remains flexible in developing a program, the student with a TBI will be provided with an appropriate program.

4. *Lack of understanding of the diagnosis of TBI.* There is often a mistaken belief that TBI refers only to the cause of the child's disability rather than to a group of children who have unique, although acquired, educational needs. When we understand these children's unique needs and their differences from other disabilities, we can appreciate the need for a separate classification.

5. *Resistance to outside sources of information.* School personnel may regard information from noneducational sources (i.e., from physicians and therapists) as unnecessary, and maybe unwanted, for their educational planning. However, information from medical personnel and therapists will help create a more comprehensive picture of the child's overall pattern of functioning.

6. *Unwillingness to begin planning prior to reentry.* School personnel may be unwilling to begin assessing and planning for a student's needs before the child returns to school, preferring instead to wait and see how the student performs in the previous class placement. As stated earlier, planning for the child's return must begin during hospitalization as it is unlikely that a child with moderate to severe injuries will return to a previous class without modification.

Hospital-to-School Transition Planning

An important step in the student's transition from the hospital to the school involves preparing school staff, parents, classmates, and the child prior to reentry.

Preparing Staff

School personnel may react in two ways to their lack of training in the area of TBI. Some feel overconfident about their ability to meet the child's needs because there are special education programs in place, whereas others panic at their lack of preparation. Both reactions, while common, are unrealistic and need to be addressed. Important realities the school staff need to accept prior to the child's reentry include (a) children with TBI demonstrate characteristics that are unique to their condition, (b) teachers and staff need to gain information that relates specifically to children with TBI, and (c) teachers and staff will be able to help the child through appropriate training.

Everyone who will be involved with the returning child should receive training about the effects of TBI. This includes the principal,

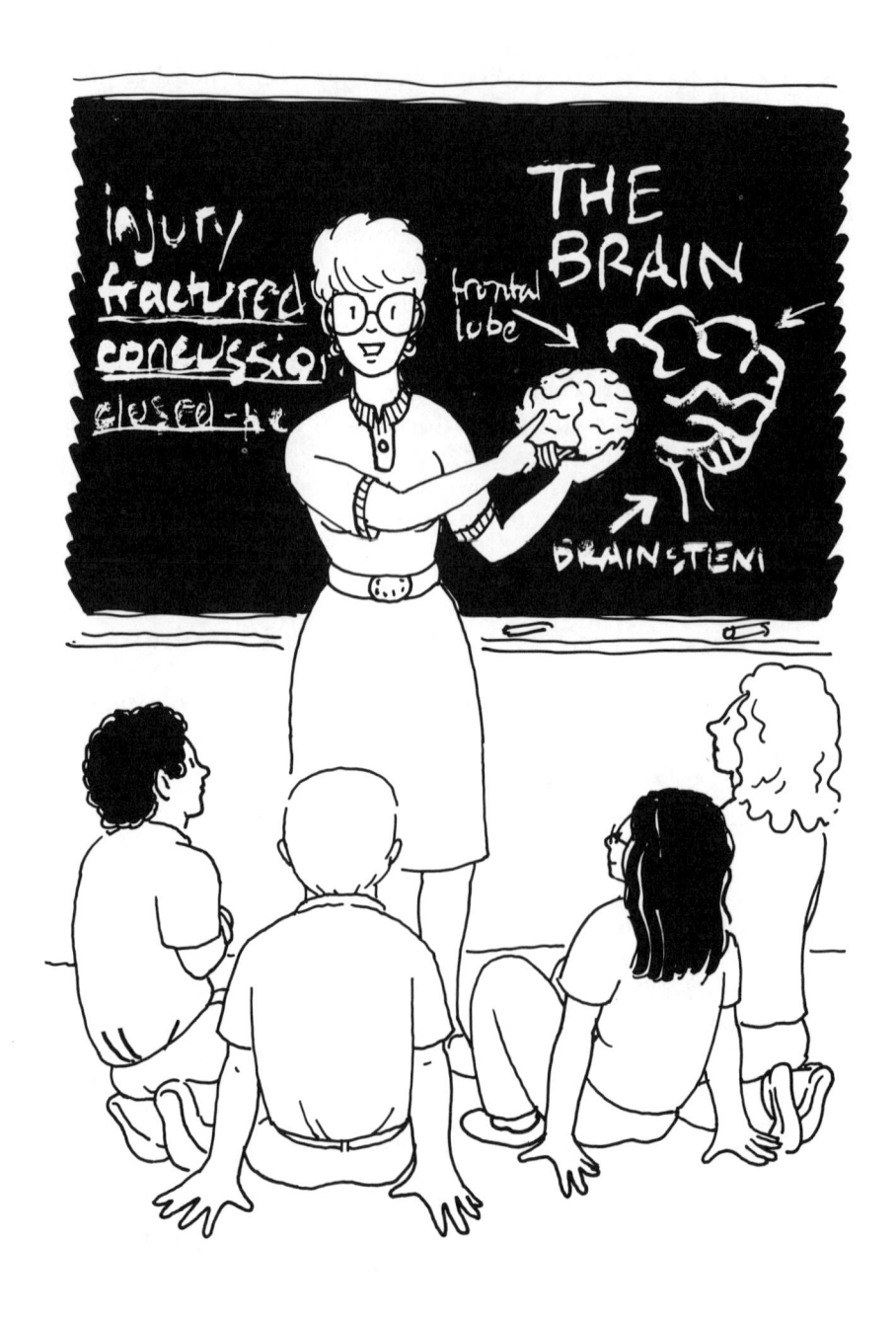

48 *Traumatic Brain Injury in Children and Adolescents*

teachers, nurses, counselors, aides, and other building workers. Such training should include the following:

- General information about the effects of TBI
- The differences between children with TBI and other handicapping conditions
- Specific information about the returning child's unique medical problems and educational needs
- The expected long-term problems the child may have
- Related services the child may need (e.g., occupational, physical, or speech therapies)
- Transition techniques for school reentry
- Instructional strategies for children with TBI
- Scheduling modifications that may be needed

This training can be conducted through inservice programs provided by the hospital rehabilitation staff, a representative of a local chapter of the National Head Injury Foundation, or specialists in the school district who are knowledgeable about TBI. The staff should also receive and review written materials that address the unique needs of students with TBI.

To further explain the recovery process, the family may choose to share with the staff any videotapes that were taken in the hospital to show the early condition of the child and demonstrate the amount of recovery that has already taken place. It is not uncommon for hospital therapy sessions (e.g., occupational or physical therapy) to be videotaped to show the child's progress.

Preparing Parents

In addition to being able to care for their child in other ways, the parents of a child with TBI need to be prepared to advocate for appropriate educational services. As soon as the child is medically stable, the parents should be given information about the long-term problems associated with TBI and the specialized educational programming their child will require. School personnel must discuss thoroughly with the family what they can expect when their child returns to school. Information parents need includes the following:

- Knowledge about the long-term effects of TBI
- Services schools are required to provide to students with disabilities
- Assessment procedures
- The process of developing an IEP

School personnel should help parents obtain this information. The National Head Injury Association or an affiliated state-level organization can also provide information and written materials on the subject.

Preparing Classmates

In preparing for the child's return to school, classmates should not be neglected. These children need to be aware that, due to an injury to the brain, their classmate may look or act differently. A general discussion about TBI and its effects will help classmates understand what happened in the injury and why the child may have changed. An open discussion allows students to ask questions and perhaps clear up rumors and other false information about the returning student. It is also helpful if the students are prepared for some of the things that may now be different or troublesome for their classmate. They should know beforehand, for example, that the child may not recall things that happened before the accident, may not remember the accident itself, and thus may not be able to answer questions about it. They should be prepared for physical changes, memory problems, speech difficulties, and any new behavioral proclivities.

Classmates should also receive specialized instructions on how to help the returning child, including how much assistance they are to give the child and when to offer assistance to the student and when not to. For example, the child may need practice in putting on a coat. Therefore, even though it looks like assistance is needed, it should not be offered. On the other hand, classmates may help the child when a special situation, such as a fire drill, occurs.

Preparing the Student with TBI

There are several ways to prepare the child for the return to school. Memory and language problems may make it difficult to explain the accident and recovery to classmates. Besides, with multiple questioning peers, the child may become frustrated by this inability to answer questions. Therefore, it is helpful if a staff member from the hospital or school helps the child plan an account of the accident and subsequent hospitalization and rehabilitation process. This account can then be presented to classmates by the child or the teacher upon return to school.

Finally, it is often helpful for the student to make brief visits to school before the actual return. Memory problems may make it difficult for the student to remember the way around the school building, for example. Brief visits enable the student to become reacquainted with the physical layout of the school building, and to have limited visits with friends and teachers. Finally, such visits may help identify physical barriers that need to be considered in the reentry planning process.

Evaluating and Modifying the School Environment

Prior to the child's reentry, the school staff must evaluate the environment to which the student will return and make necessary adjustments to accommodate the child's unique characteristics. The following are several general questions that should be considered prior to reentry.

1. *What is the best setting in which to provide the child's instruction?* The returning child's cognitive deficits often necessitate one-to-one instruction. While group settings help provide needed social interaction and skills, attention and concentration problems often limit the usefulness of group instruction in the early stages. With one-to-one instruction, the teacher is able to refocus the child's attention as soon as it wanders. As the child's concentration improves, additional students may be added to the instructional session.

2. *How structured does the environment need to be?* Generally, the student requires much more structure than is generally offered in the regular classroom. Distracting stimuli must be reduced; room changes need to be kept at a minimum. Even at the high school level, the student may require that classroom rules and expectations be well structured, frequently reviewed, and perhaps even posted.

3. *How much organization needs to be added to the program?* Because of temporal and spatial deficits after TBI, the returning student may require additional organizational features in the educational program. For example, someone may need to be assigned to assist

the child in reviewing the day's schedule and help organize the material needed for the day or for a particular class. Specific periods may be scheduled in a resource room, where the student can review with the special instructor what will be happening during the day, what the assignments have been, and what material needs to be taken home that evening.

4. *What instructional devices must be available to the student on return to school?* Because of physical and/or cognitive problems, the student may require supplemental devices to complete assignments. For example, a computer may be helpful for word processing for the student who has difficulty producing written material. Similarly, a calculator may be used by those who understand the multiplication process, but have difficulty remembering the multiplication facts. A reading guide (e.g., a straight edge) can help students who have difficulty keeping their place on the page.

Furthermore, computer software programs can supplement instruction by providing drill and practice for a variety of skills. In particular, programs that do not impose time restraints are suitable for the child with a TBI.

For some students, the speech therapist may have recommended devices to augment communication. To ensure a smooth transition, either needed equipment should be available in the school or plans must be made for transporting equipment that the student uses in therapy or at home.

School Calendar and Daily Scheduling

The timing of a student's return to school must not be fortuitous, but should be carefully planned. One child, for whom reentry planning had not been carried out, surprised the teachers by being returned to school on Halloween for the first time following a TBI. His mother erroneously thought that this would be a good way for him to feel positive about his return. In reality, the boy was agitated by the excessive stimuli and by the novelty of the occasion, and became quickly fatigued by all the activity and needed to be precipitously returned home.

Adjustments in the child's school schedule are often required to help compensate for the child's physical and mental limitations, and to provide needed cognitive stimulation. Such adjustments may include a shortened school day, scheduling modifications, and year-round instruction. Because children with TBI need continual cognitive stimulation, they often require instruction throughout the summer months. If summer classes are not available, homebound services can provide the student with instruction during the summer months.

Because children with TBI often experience significant fatigue, the student may be able to attend school for only part of the day or may require a modified schedule to allow for several in-school rest periods. The time the child spends in school should be lengthened gradually as physical and cognitive capabilities increase.

During the school day, the schedule should be structured so that taxing academic subjects are taken early in the day when the child is most alert. In addition, to provide necessary breaks, study periods or individual work periods with the resource teacher may be scheduled throughout the day.

IEP Planning

School personnel often lack experience in developing programs for children with TBI. Translating information from a variety of sources and disciplines is not easy. However, some general guidelines will aid educators in designing a program that will meet the child's educational needs.

As with any child, when developing an IEP for the child with a TBI, the following general questions need to be addressed:

1. What are the current levels of the student's cognitive functioning?
2. How has the TBI affected the child's language, motor skills, self-concept, social development, and academic achievement?
3. Given the student's current needs, what is the most appropriate service delivery system?
4. What are realistic goals for the student?
5. How can the school, family, and community provide sound support for optimum recovery?
6. What residual physical or medical problems are likely to interfere with functioning in the educational setting?
7. How can residual physical problems be addressed?

After answering these questions and determining the child's needs, an IEP can be developed. Great flexibility must be exercised in developing this plan, with major attention to the child's overall needs. Therefore, goals such as improving attention to task, following directions, or increasing language skills are more appropriate for the student with TBI than such goals as learning math facts or spelling words. Because many teachers are accustomed to writing goals that address highly specific deficit areas, it may be difficult for them to obtain an overall view of the child's functioning and address the more global deficits for the student with TBI.

Case Management

To effectively coordinate the many people and all the procedures involved in a well-executed reentry plan, it is useful to include a case management component. A *case manager* serves as liaison among school, family, and rehabilitation professionals; assures that all are informed about the child's progress and needs; and performs many tasks that assure a coordinated transition from hospital, through reentry, to school. The roles of the case manager may include those described below.

Communication Link

The case manager begins communicating with the hospital or rehabilitation facility while the student is still hospitalized and arranges observations by school personnel of the child's rehabilitation therapies. By being in touch with key rehabilitation staff, the case manager keeps educators informed of the child's progress, while providing the rehabilitation staff with information about the student's prior functioning and the resources available in the school. Appendix C includes a checklist of activities that a school case manager may request from hospital staff during the child's hospitalization.

The case manager may invite family and rehabilitation staff to the school to help assess the setting both before and after reentry to help ensure that barriers to effective reentry are not overlooked. As a vital communication link, the case manager needs to be an alert troubleshooter, who recognizes when family or educator stress may be alleviated by paying attention to the information exchange among everyone.

Meeting Convener and Moderator

The case manager may encourage joint meetings between rehabilitation and school staff as scheduled treatment and discharge conferences are planned. Many times, educators are not involved in these important information exchanges, not because they are not welcome, but because the rehabilitation staff did not think to include them due to limited experience with schools.

The case manager may be the one to convene the educational conferences in the school. A very important role is that of ensuring that those involved in the child's education meet relatively frequently (at least monthly at first) to review progress and make needed revisions.

Translator

Hospital and therapy records may contain a wealth of information about the child's functioning and needs. Often such material is available in a form that is minimally useful to educators. For example, information about how long a child was comatose may lie handwritten only in the ICU chart notes. Similarly, indications of the depth of family concern or distress may be found in nursing records. A trained case manager who has had experience working with returning children with TBI will know sources of information within the medical system, will know how to follow approved procedures to gather all such relevant data, and will be able to translate this material for school planning. For example, it is extremely helpful for educators if the case manager obtains the hospital discharge summaries prepared by the physician in charge.

In addition to gathering all necessary information, the case manager may draft a document that is functional for schools by preparing an integrated summary of all of the reports, giving an overview of significant features of the child's injury, progress in therapy, and continued needs (see sample summary in Appendix D). For example, the hospital physical therapist may note that the child has significant problems of balance and motor planning, and has difficulty transitioning from one position to another. Throughout, the record may contain notes about the child's dangerous impulsivity, poor judgment, and lack of emotional control. The case manager's integrated report will inform the members of the planning team that because of poor balance and impulse control, the child may make quick, thoughtless moves that may lead to loss of balance and a fall. Therefore, the student will need assistance getting up and will be angry about accepting help.

Information Resource for Family and School

The case manager may be responsible for maintaining up-to-date medical records, evaluation reports, and educational planning reports. After the student is discharged from the hospital, this task may involve maintaining records relating to outpatient follow-ups and therapies, and compiling for the school a list of agencies and professionals important for this student.

The case manager will also be available to families for information sharing or for answering questions about educational procedures. In addition, this person may be able to alert families to relevant community resources, such as local or state programs affiliated with the National Head Injury Foundation and local family support groups.

Inservice Coordinator

The case manager may be the one to arrange for inservice programs for teachers, administrators, and other school personnel, as well as for classmates, so that everyone involved has knowledge about TBI and knows what to expect when the student returns. An experienced case manager may be the person to conduct such inservice for the school.

The case manager role may be assumed by a variety of school professionals, including school psychologists, counselors, social workers, or special education administrators. Some school districts have a specially trained person, perhaps a staff member who has volunteered for the role, who is designated case manager for all students with TBI in that district. Although the list of duties appears formidable, a professional with knowledge of TBI and experience in case management will find this role both interesting and rewarding.

Summary

School Preparation

- Provide for student's safety
- Inform all school staff
- Determine appropriate program intensity and structure

- Procure special equipment
- Design behavior management program
- Define community resources
- Define staff communication procedures and intervals

Barriers

- Uninformed staff
- Inflexible programming
- Resistance to unfamiliar information resources
- Reluctance to initiate preentry planning

Roles of the Case Manager

- Communicates with rehabilitation facility
- Arranges meetings between school and rehabilitation staff
- Translates medical information for educators
- Provides information about TBI to family and educators
- Coordinates school inservice programs

8
Assessment of the Student with Traumatic Brain Injury

The assessment process is an important step in educational planning for all students with disabilities; however, several considerations are unique to those returning to school following a TBI. First, the evaluation for the purposes of school planning is set in a context of ongoing assessment which begins while the child is still in acute hospital care and ideally continues for several years. Second, the assessment involves evaluation strategies and methods that differ from the usual special education testing. Third, special educators must often rely on evaluation data generated outside of the school evaluation. The comprehensiveness of material provided to the school and the expertise of the school evaluation team dictate the degree to which the team integrates these data into their evaluations.

Longitudinal Nature of Assessment

Although the amount of damage to the brain affects the degree of subsequent cognitive impairment, there is not a direct relationship between the regions of the brain that are injured and the degree and type of resulting cognitive deficits. Therefore, the primary way to determine the pattern of cognitive strengths and deficits is to conduct a comprehensive neuropsychological assessment. Also, the information provided is critical to planning an appropriate program for the child.

The rehabilitation staff working with the child begin to survey the child's functioning early in the postinjury period. For example, the child's ability to understand and express language, to focus and sustain attention, to recall factual and new information, and to remember events of the day are monitored almost daily. When the child is able to attend for 10–15 minutes, respond to instructions, and develop a continuous memory for a day's events, an initial neuropsychological assessment should take place. The findings from this evaluation should be used by those planning the child's reentry.

Importance of a Neuropsychological Examination

Several important benefits are derived from a thorough neuropsychological examination.

1. *It provides a comprehensive picture of all cognitive functions that are vital for learning.* The behavior and learning characteristics the student brings to the classroom are the result of the functioning of the entire brain. The neuropsychological evaluation systematically assesses the entire range of behaviors subsumed by the brain. Because a TBI results in widespread damage, it affects both basic and higher level functions. Educators need to know all of the student's abilities, as each affects how the student will learn in relation to age expectations and how the student will function adaptively.

All too often, children return to school following a TBI before educators have formed a complete picture of the children's abilities. For students in the early grades, in particular, mere reacquisition of previous skills is often mistaken for rapid learning. The child's deficits are not recognized until new learning is required.

2. *A neuropsychological assessment aids in predicting outcome.* This is particularly important for younger children in whom the effects will not be evident until later years. Therefore, a systematic evaluation of all cognitive foundations for learning is the only way in which we can identify what the later deficits may be.

3. *Neuropsychological assessment aids educators in selecting programming and remediation targets.* The evaluation results pro-

vide information about the child's present functioning in relation to age expectations and define the pattern of residual deficits and strengths.

Components of a Neuropsychological Evaluation

The neuropsychological evaluation provides information about the following areas of functioning:

- Cognitive/intellectual
- Sensory and perceptual
- Motor and psychomotor
- Language
- Visual spatial/constructional
- Memory
- Higher level problem solving

Additionally, a neuropsychological examination conducted by a professional trained in TBI can reveal deficits in the foundation skills that are often impaired after a TBI. A problem in any of these skills significantly affects performance of more complex skills and ability to learn, but may not be apparent on cursory examination. Thus, the evaluation can be valuable by providing the special educator with information about these abilities, including the following:

- Focusing and sustaining attention
- Reaction time in physical and mental tasks
- Memory for old and new material
- Organizing information
- Use of feedback
- Information processing
- Problem solving, flexibility in selecting new strategies, anticipating consequences, and planning ahead
- Holding several pieces of information in mind simultaneously while problem solving

- Generating hypotheses
- Self-initiative in problem solving
- Awareness of performance adequacy
- Functioning in the facet of novel versus familiar tasks
- Dealing with stress of difficult tasks

Although a neuropsychological assessment provides important information about the student's cognitive pattern, it shares limitations with other evaluation tools. For example, decisions about the student's qualitative features are as dependent on examiner sophistication as on other measures. Also, the results are obtained in a one-to-one standardized setting, whereas educators need to know how the student will use the skills in the classroom and the wide community.

Differences Between Neuropsychological and Other Evaluations

A comprehensive neuropsychological evaluation differs from a typical psychological assessment in the range of abilities studied. It differs also in the selection of cognitive factors viewed as important for program planning. Intelligence tests alone are not sufficient to determine the cognitive deficits of children with TBI. Although the *Wechsler Intelligence Scale for Children–Revised* or the *Wechsler Adult Intelligence Scale–Revised* is a pivotal component of many neuropsychological batteries, an intelligence test by itself is not sensitive to all of the cognitive sequelae. A single IQ test neither examines memory, attention, and organizational functions, nor adequately portrays deficits in the foundation skills, which may have major effects on new learning. Appendix E presents the evaluation report of a student still in the early postinjury stage whose many cognitive deficits would not have been adequately understood based on a single measure.

The way in which educators use psychometric data also differs for children with TBI. Whereas for many special education students, intelligence test results are used to determine eligibility for special educational services, such use is not appropriate for children with TBI. Although severely injured students may score within the range of retardation, their characteristics and programming needs differ in many ways from those of students with developmental retardation. Also, the IQ–achievement discrepancy, used for defining eligibility for services for learning disability, for example, is not an appropriate consideration for students with TBI. In the period shortly after the injury, these children's IQ scores may still be depressed and achievement scores may not yet reflect problems with new learning. Thus, although they may suffer marked disabilities in new learning, students with TBI do not share psychometric characteristics of children classified as learning disabled.

Another way in which the assessment needs of children with TBI differ from those of other students in special education derives from rapid changes in their cognitive characteristics in the first year after injury. Thus, they require more frequent assessment to avoid basing programming on outdated information. It is recommended that children with TBI receive comprehensive assessments at 6-month intervals for the first year after injury.

Neuropsychological Batteries

To evaluate a child following a TBI, a neuropsychologist uses a battery of tests that tap the range of significant cognitive variables. A common battery is based on the Halstead–Reitan tests. The adult battery (Reitan & Wolfson, 1985) may be used with students over age 14. Another form of the battery provides instructions, tasks, and norms for children of ages 9–14 (Reitan & Davison, 1974). Finally, an adaptation based on the downward scaling and substitution of tests is available for children between ages 5 and 8 (Reitan, 1969). These batteries evaluate a range of functions:

- Sensory perceptual abilities in tactile, auditory, and visual modalities
- Appreciation of the basic phonological aspects of language
- Verbal and nonverbal memory
- Motor efficiency for simple as well as complex psychomotor tasks
- Lateral dominance
- Ability to use feedback and learn under novel conditions
- Flexibility in problem solving

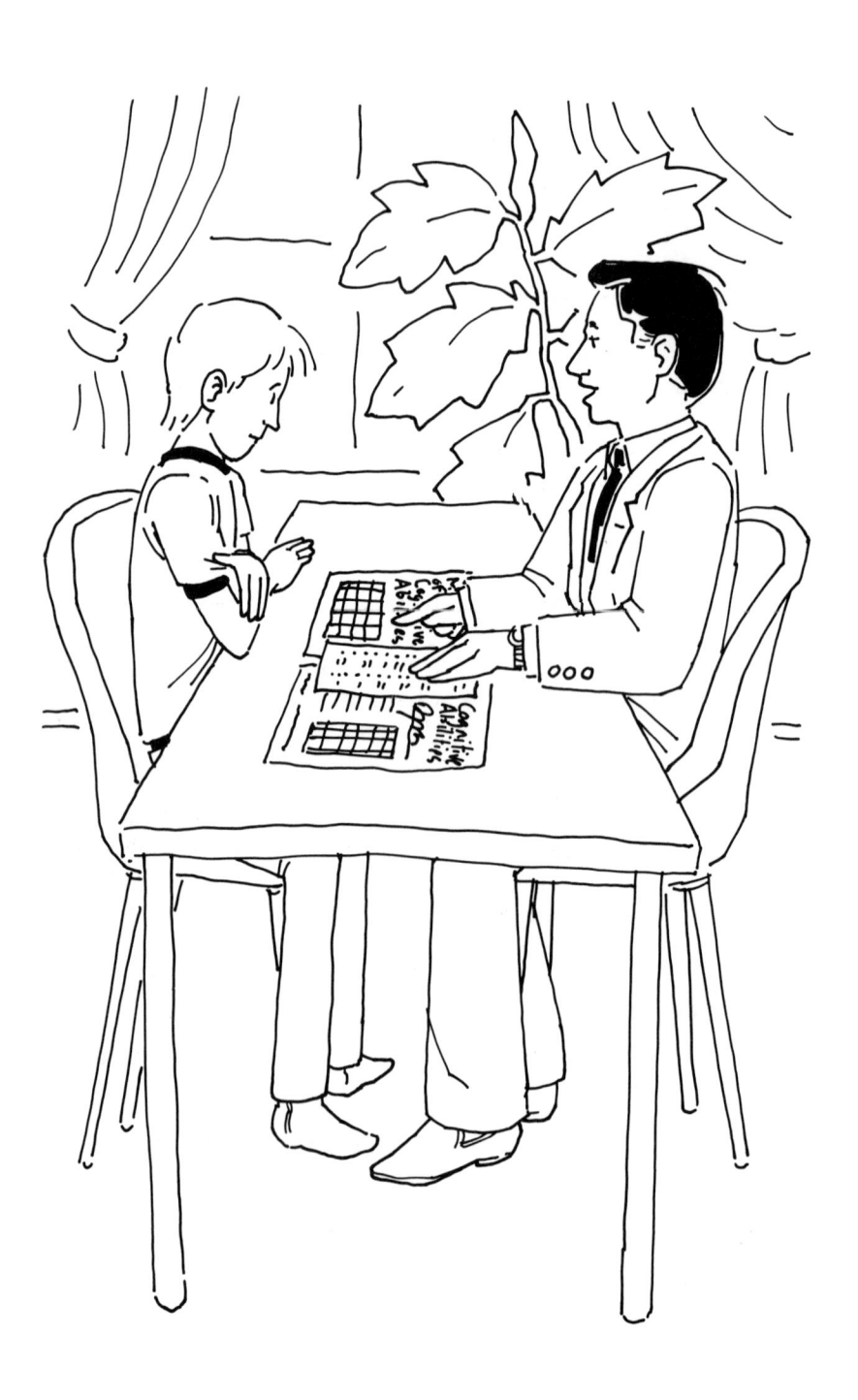

Understanding Neuropsychological Findings

It is to the advantage of students with TBI and the school planning teams to have access to the findings of the neuropsychological evaluation and the current findings from the child's therapists at the time of reentry planning. The ease with which these data are translated into programming recommendations rests on several factors:

1. The familiarity of the neuropsychologist and the rehabilitation team with educational possibilities and realities
2. The sophistication of school staff knowledge about TBI
3. The availability of a consultant in TBI or a case manager who can bridge the gap between those who have evaluated and treated the child during the acute period and special educators who will plan for the child

A common concern expressed by teachers is that neuropsychological reports prepared outside of the school do not easily translate into classroom instruction. There are several ways in which teachers can get assistance in translating the findings. The teacher can talk directly with the neuropsychologist who prepared the report, or members of the school team who are knowledgeable in areas of neuropsychology and/or TBI can assist in interpreting the findings. By including the neuropsychologist in the staffings at the school, there is potential for greater communication for the benefit of the student.

Schools are responding to the need for greater staff skills in TBI in a variety of ways. Some large districts, which may serve many children with TBI, have trained a designated team that serves all children in the district with TBI. Also, as schools become more alert to the special needs of children with TBI, special educators, school psychologists, and therapists are seeking competency in TBI and neuropsychological assessment. Collaboration between special educators and rehabilitation specialists in TBI also is becoming more frequent. This allows rehabilitation specialists, particularly neuropsychologists, to learn more about the kinds of information special educators need, and it helps educators to develop sophistication about TBI.

Implications of Neuropsychological Deficits for Classroom Functioning

The sample neuropsychological evaluation report presented in Appendix E gives several examples of identified deficits that have implications for how the child will handle learning in the classroom. A few other examples follow.

Problems with sustained attention and concentration have significant consequences for new learning. The student will have problems concentrating on classroom work and homework, be easily distracted, and experience difficulty following instructions and shifting attention from one instructional task to another.

Difficulty committing new information to memory also has grave consequences and, as with attention difficulty, is almost continuously interfering. The student will not recall assignments, or even that an assignment was made; will not be able to return to a task if interrupted; and will be limited when learning new facts or procedures.

Problems with visual spatial reasoning not only will show up on paper-and-pencil tasks, but may impair the student's ability to navigate within the school building, locate sections of a book, and interpret nonverbal facial and gestural communication cues.

Problems with organization will affect classroom skills such as summarizing, outlining, and separating the most relevant facts from a body of information. Problems with speeded output or response time for manual activities may mean that the student cannot keep up with dictated work, will need more time to copy assignments from the board, or will perform poorly on tests because of an inability to get to all of the questions. Slow mental processing may cause the student to appear inept and unable to answer a question. As a result, quicker peers may leave the student behind in conversations. Even deficits in perceiving tactile information will interfere as the student fumbles with a locker key or combination.

When educators possess this kind of comprehensive information at the time of reentry planning, both the student and teachers benefit. Teachers can anticipate areas of difficulty and design a program to accommodate them, and the student returns to a program that is appropriate for the new learning needs.

Summary

Functions Tapped by a Neuropsychological Evaluation

- Cognitive/intellectual
- Sensory and perceptual
- Motor and psychomotor

- Language
- Visual spatial/constructional
- Memory
- Higher level problem solving

How Neuropsychological Evaluation Differs from Typical Assessment

- Wider range of functions assessed
- Cognitive factors viewed as important for programming
- IQ–achievement discrepancy determination not the goal

9

Programming for Students with Traumatic Brain Injury

After planning for reentry, devising a schedule, and modifying the environment, educators need to develop programming strategies to meet the child's specialized needs. Unfortunately, no standard procedures or curricula are available specifically for students with TBI. Instead, school personnel need to develop methods for teaching the child based on the information obtained during the assessment process.

The child's cognitive, language, and attention deficits will need direct remediation. Therefore, cognitive retraining activities are required. Specific deficits (e.g., auditory discrimination problems or a restricted visual field) demand specific strategies for remediation. This chapter provides a description of cognitive retraining and a list of common deficit areas with suggestions for specific strategies for how to remediate the problems.

Cognitive Retraining Within the School

Special educators who teach students with TBI will encounter the terms *cognitive rehabilitation*, *retraining*, or *remediation*. Sometimes used interchangeably, such terms refer to the treatment of the cognitively based deficits associated with TBI. The goal is to improve post-TBI functioning more than would occur by spontaneous recovery.

Cognitive rehabilitation varies widely in terms of what its focus is, who conducts it, and where it is implemented. For some professionals, cognitive rehabilitation means treatment to restore functions to a previous level by directly training the impaired cognitive skills. Others, more realistically, view its goals as enhancing residual cognitive skills so the child can function as effectively as possible. Cognitive retraining in a rehabilitation setting may be conducted by neuropsychologists or may be incorporated into the treatment programs of speech, occupational, and recreational therapists.

In terms of location, cognitive retraining or rehabilitation may be delivered in isolation from the rest of the child's daily activities, such as in an individual treatment session in a separate therapy room. In this setting, the child may get one-to-one training, possibly via computer-presented attention, vigilance, or memory tasks. However, it is becoming increasingly apparent that cognitive rehabilitation cannot be divorced from the mainstream of the child's daily life; therefore, it is more effective when incorporated into functional activities.

The Educator's Role in Cognitive Retraining

Educators should not be awed by the mystique associated with the concept of cognitive retraining. The most successful cognitive retraining takes place in settings where functional skills are applied. The school is an ideal setting, therefore, because it is in the classroom that the impact of the child's deficits show up. The school will play a major role in cognitive retraining because the child's deficits can be remediated in the context in which they occur. Thus, cognitive processes such as attention, memory, and thought organization skills can be redeveloped and enhanced, and such skills as developing judgment, problem solving, planning for the future, retention, organizing/integrating input, comprehending detail, word retrieval, abstract reasoning, and analysis skills can all be remediated in the classroom.

Specialized materials are not needed to carry out cognitive retraining in the school setting. Instead, the regular academic curriculum and daily activities serve as the basis. To develop specific skills, the child's own schoolwork can be adapted to the current level of functioning. For example, to address the student's comprehension problems, the teacher can use class material or the daily newspapers for developing learning activities to help the student identify the main idea in a story or locate sentences containing answers. The teacher can help the student work on memory deficits by using activities such as following directions, rapid retrieval exercises, and silent reading for details. For improving judgment, the teacher can use activities that require the child to respond to a given social situation or plan how to carry out a complex activity (e.g., giving a party). To aid problem-solving skills, math word problems, devising a class schedule, or planning routes using maps can be used. For organization and sequencing skills, the child can be required to write a multistep cartoon, plan a worldwide tour, or list the steps needed to carry out some other complex activity.

The classroom computer can also be a useful tool in cognitive retraining. Drill-and-practice computer programs are helpful in developing and redeveloping skills of children with TBI, especially programs that emphasize memory skills or problem solving skills. Furthermore, organization and sequencing skills can be practiced by having the child set up the computer for use.

Cognitive retraining activities should be carried out in a variety of situations and should include both individual and group tasks. Providing as much practice as possible, in as many settings as possible, will help the student to generalize skills.

Programming for Specific Deficits

Assessment information provided by hospital or school personnel can be used to develop programming strategies. The following is a listing of some common deficit areas and suggested techniques for dealing with them.

- Auditory discrimination
  - Ensure that background noise is minimal (e.g., room dividers can be used to help reduce room noise).
  - Provide preferential seating to enable the student to get the maximum benefits from both auditory and visual cues.
  - Gain the student's attention before speaking and check to make sure the student has understood what was discussed.
  - Provide a study area relatively free of auditory distractions for the student to use when completing assignments.

- Restricted visual field
  - Teach the student to use verbal cues such as "look all the way to the right and left" to ensure complete scanning of visual fields.
  - Ask the student to move the hand from one side of the paper to the other as a physical reminder to look at all the writing on the page.
  - Teach the student proper positioning of materials to achieve optimal visual fields.
- Maintaining attention
  - Provide a study carrel or preferential seating.
  - After giving instructions, check for proper attention and understanding by having the student repeat them.
  - Teach the student to use self-regulating techniques to maintain attention (e.g., asking "Am I paying attention?" "What is the required task?").
- Memory
  - Teach the student to use external aides such as notes, memos, daily schedule sheets, and assignment sheets.
  - Use visual imagery, when possible, to supplement oral content.
  - Teach visual imaging techniques for information presented.
  - Teach strategies for organizing information and retrieving contextual material.
  - Provide repetition and frequent review of instruction materials.
  - Provide immediate and frequent feedback to enable the student to interpret success or failure.
- Following directions
  - Provide the student with both visual and auditory directions.
  - Model tasks, whenever possible.
  - Break multistep directions into small parts and list them so that the student can refer back when needed.
  - For complex directions such as those required for a project, tape record directions and allow the student to listen to them as many times as is necessary.

PROGRAMMING **73**

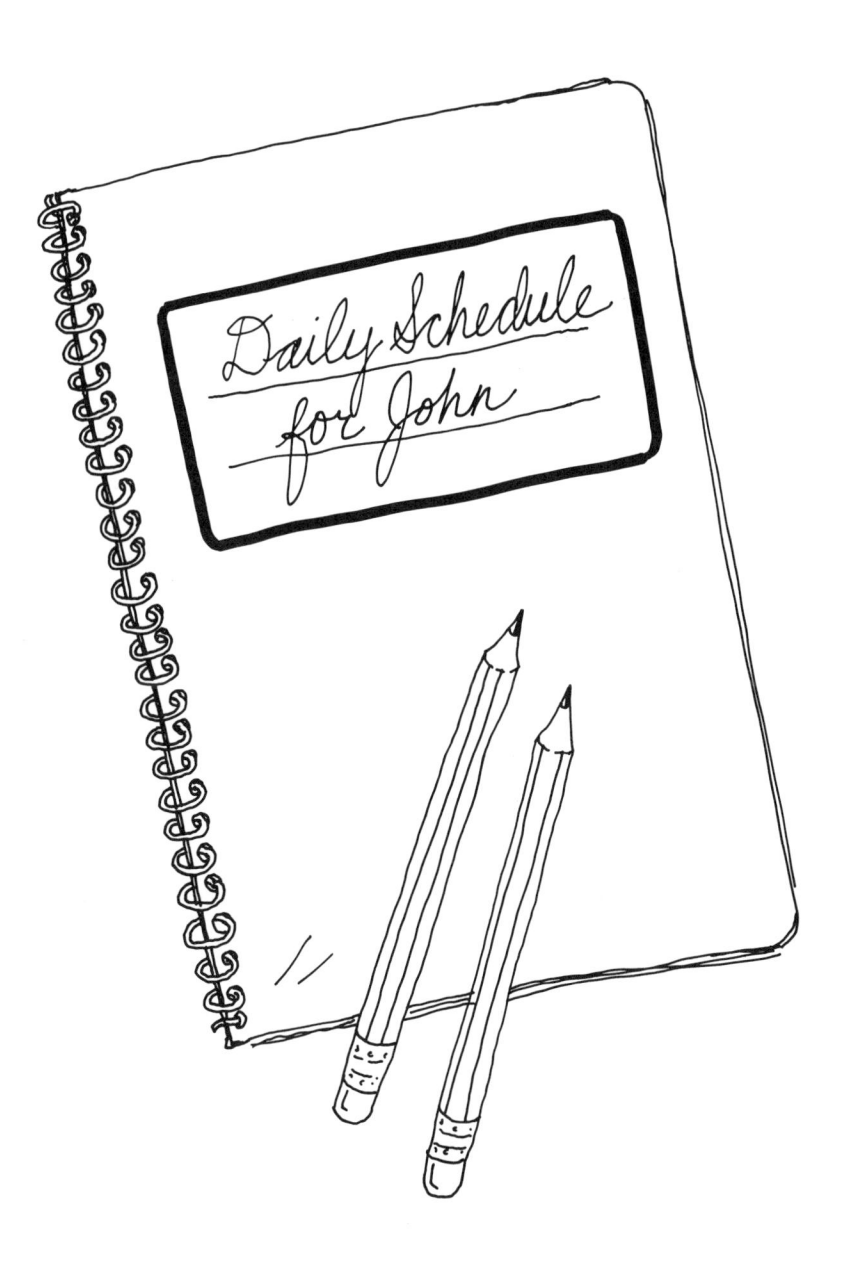

- Receptive language
  - Limit the amount of information presented at one time.
  - Provide simple instructions for only one activity at a time.
  - Have the student repeat instructions.
  - Go over practice examples, and ask the student to demonstrate ability to do the task.
  - Use concrete language.
  - Teach the student to ask the speaker to slow down, repeat, or clarify information when necessary.
- Expressive language
  - Teach the student to rehearse silently before verbally replying.
  - Teach the student to look for cues from listeners to ascertain that the student is being understood.
  - Teach the student to directly ask if he or she is being understood.
- Impulsiveness
  - Teach the student to mentally rehearse steps before beginning an activity.
  - Reduce potential distractions.
  - Frequently restate and reinforce rules.
- Problem solving
  - Have the student generate possible solutions to problems as they arise in an activity.
  - Teach the student the steps involved in problem solving (e.g., identify the problem, list relevant information, evaluate possible solutions, create an action plan).
- Slow processing
  - Allow the student additional time to process information and complete tasks.
  - Provide sufficient time for the student to respond to verbal questioning.
  - Reduce work requirements (e.g., ask the student to complete 20 of the 40 math problems).

- Have the student take exams in settings that do not have time constraints.
- Motor skills
  - Allow the student to complete a project rather than turn in a written assignment.
  - Have the student use a typewriter or a word processor to complete assignments.
  - Allow extra time for completing tasks requiring fine-motor skills.
  - Assign someone to take notes for the student during lectures.
  - Allow the student to use a dictaphone or tape recorder for copying lengthy assignments from the board.
- Lack of motivation
  - Videotape the student's classroom performance to allow the child to see improvements in functioning over a period of weeks.
  - Have the student graph his or her performance on a particular task.
  - Save samples of the student's written work over a period of time to show improvements.
- Lack of effective strategies
  - Teach strategies for reading content-area material.
  - Teach the student how to take notes during lectures.
  - Provide strategies for studying for and taking exams.
  - To help compensate for memory difficulties, teach the student to keep lists or reminder notes.
  - Provide assignment sheets to aid recall of individual class assignments.
  - Teach the student strategies for self-monitoring attention.
- General modifications for assignments
  - Record reading assignments so the student can listen while following the text.
  - Adapt text by highlighting the most important passages.
  - Provide a written set of questions before reading the material so the student knows what information to focus on.

— Ask directive questions so that the student recognizes important points.

Dealing with Behavior Problems

As stated previously, behavior problems are the result of several factors. Regardless of origin, however, these problems need to be managed. If behavior problems are programmed for and specifically dealt with, improvements can be made in the child's functioning.

1. *Help the child understand deficits* (e.g., memory or attention problems). Many behavior problems arise because the child is unaware of or unable to understand the deficits. By helping the child to recognize them, the teacher may show the child how to compensate for or readjust to lost skills.

2. *Include the child in groups with other children who have disabilities.* As a result of the deficits that stem from a TBI, children often may feel withdrawn or isolated. To encourage adjustment, it may be beneficial for the child to be included in group discussions with other children who have suffered a TBI or have handicapping conditions that set them apart from other children.

3. *Teach the child appropriate behavior.* Behavior problems may occur because judgment deficits do not allow the child to understand what constitutes appropriate behavior. Impaired judgment leads the child to do things that teachers and peers find annoying. For example, one adolescent boy teased and joked with teachers in the same manner he did with his friends. Because of social perception problems, he did not understand that it was acceptable to joke with peers, but not to act the same way toward teachers. By pointing out to a child what constitutes appropriate behavior, modeling this behavior, and reinforcing the behavior, a teacher can help the child learn appropriate behaviors.

4. *Provide direct social skills training.* Behavior problems may occur because the child has forgotten how to interact with others. Social skills training may begin with one-to-one interactions, followed by small group situations that require limited interactions. After the child has demonstrated progress in those situations, the student can be placed in large group settings that require cooperation among students. In these settings, students can be taught to take turns in conversational interchanges, display appropriate behavior, and look for cues from others to evaluate their own performance.

5. *Use time-out when necessary.* Occasionally, the student may become extremely noncompliant, making removal from the environment necessary. It is also beneficial for children to learn to identify their own frustration level before it escalates to extremes.

Educators should discuss behavior problems with persons from the child's rehabilitation setting, to obtain realistic expectations for the child's behavior. Rehabilitation staff can also share techniques they have found useful for dealing with the child's behavior. It may also be helpful for teachers to consult with district personnel who specialize in behavior management techniques. These consultants help design specific behavior management programs that take into account a child's deficits. Finally, teachers should explain behavior management techniques to parents and work with parents to gain the needed support in developing a behavior management program that will be carried out in school as well as at home.

Teacher Reactions to the Long-Term Effects of TBI

In the beginning stages, teachers may be amazed at how quickly the child is able to return to school, in spite of the seriousness of the child's accident and the length of the coma. Knowing the details of the child's initial medical condition, teachers are often overjoyed by how well the child seems to be recovering. Thus, comments such as, "Just a few weeks ago he was in a coma, but now he is doing so well that he is able to walk and talk again," are not uncommon because physical recovery is erroneously equated with overall recovery. Often, when the child first returns to school, long-term cognitive problems are overlooked by those focusing on the child's rapid physical gains.

In addition, when the child returns to school, many concessions may have been made to program for specific needs, making it possible for the child to perform successfully, without revealing true deficits. However, satisfactory performance in such a program does not mean that the child can return to the regular class and to previous levels. It is important to remember that the reason the child is doing so well is that the program is tailored to the student's needs.

When the child appears to be doing well in a modified program, it is tempting for teachers to want to intensify the child's program by adding more classes. The student may even ask to take more classes or to be removed from a resource room because things are going well. Teachers want students to be involved in planning their programs, know their capabilities, and make decisions about their own stamina and fitness; however, as we have emphasized, following TBI, students may not be able to accurately assess their abilities.

Another common reaction is for teachers to question their own teaching skills. Thus, if the child fails to meet unrealistic expectations, teachers may attribute this to their inability to find the right way to teach the child.

Sources of Teacher Frustration

It is not uncommon for teachers to become frustrated when working with students who have TBI. Progress, although rapid in the early period, may slow to the point where the student seems to be making no progress at all. Teachers may become frustrated with the child's lack of learning and their own inability to teach the child. Lacking well-prescribed methods and training materials for children with TBI, teachers may feel they do not know what to do.

Another source of teacher frustration derives from the child's normal appearance despite continued deficits. As a result, teachers forget that the child's erratic behavior and learning problems are a result of a head injury and require special interventions and programming modifications. To avoid some of the frustrations teachers typically experience when working with a student who has a TBI, the following suggestions may help:

1. Obtain as much knowledge as possible about TBI, especially long-term outcomes.
2. Know the child's specific deficits.
3. Do not equate physical recovery with overall recovery.
4. Do not lose sight of deficits as the child begins to pick up old skills and starts to appear to be functioning normally.
5. Clearly lay out behavioral and instructional expectations. Do not assume that the child knows what is expected.
6. Understand what triggers problem behaviors. If the child acts out because of frustration, adaptations in programming are probably required.
7. Do not give students major responsibility for making decisions about programming if they demonstrate deficits in judgment and

reasoning. Such deficits preclude them from fully understanding their own needs.

Community Responses to Long-Standing Effects

Following a traumatic injury, especially in a small community, people may be aware of the child's accident and offer support and encouragement. When the child first gets out of the hospital, people are aware of what caused the child's physical disabilities and may go out of their way to offer assistance. However, problems sometimes arise from people who are unaware that the physical problems are due to an injury. For example, persons who did not know about the accident may accuse the child of drinking or being on drugs because of abnormal gait.

Following physical recovery, people will expect the child to function normally. A lack of understanding of underlying language and memory problems may cause individuals to think the child is "stupid" when unable to give directions, to provide the proper change when making a purchase, or to carry on a coherent conversation. They may hire adolescents with TBI for a summer job they are capable of performing, only to fire them later because they are unable to keep up with the work.

The common reactions of teachers and the community generally stem from a lack of knowledge about the long-term effects of TBI. This lack of understanding often adds to the child's feelings of frustration and lack of self-worth. Being aware of what the student may experience will help teachers gain a better understanding of the problems faced by the student with a TBI.

The School's Role in Students' Career/Life Planning

Because many head injuries happen to adolescents in their junior and senior years of high school, the implications for career/life planning are significant. Most students with TBI are unwilling to consider the benefits of delaying graduation while benefiting from the education system's provisions for vocational training until age 22, and opt for pursuing high school graduation on time with classmates.

Stories abound about teenagers who returned to school after a head injury and managed to complete course requirements in time to graduate with their class. Those who went away to college to pursue their pre-TBI career aspirations often were unable to complete even the first semester. At this point, the public education system was no longer responsible because these students had already graduated from high school. Many do not find financial resources or specialized post–high school programs to develop skills to enter the job market successfully.

Fortunately, many community colleges are developing programs to provide additional vocational training to students with TBI. Modified courses and counselors knowledgeable about the effects of head injury are also becoming available on many community college campuses and in some universities.

In some cases, state vocational rehabilitation agencies provide post–high school training. Their services include aptitude assessment, training opportunities for developing independent living skills, and supervised trial job placement. In addition, they can assist with modifying equipment for the employer, the student, or both, and can provide funds for extended training at vocational schools or community colleges.

To take advantage of these services, the crucial first step is for the student to complete an application. Therefore, high school counselors need to be aware of and informed about the range of opportunities vocational rehabilitation agencies offer. This information, in turn, will enable them to encourage and direct the student with TBI to needed services.

Follow-up studies have shown unemployment rates of 70% among previously employed adults with TBI (Brooks, McKinlay, Symington, Beattie, & Campsie, 1987). Such figures show the dramatic reduction of a survivor's ability to compete for jobs in the marketplace.

Once again, schools have a clear responsibility to provide students with TBI reasonable alternatives to graduation by age 18. Unfortunately, most educators believe in the self-determination potential of maturing young people and are reluctant to intervene in the student's strong push for graduation. Too late, it becomes apparent that the student's lack of self-awareness poses a major threat to completing a college education.

As educators become more knowledgeable about head injury, they will devise various ways, which are socially acceptable to the student, to delay official graduation until viable career/life alternatives are clearer. Students with TBI need to select an occupation based on realistic self-appraisal of strengths and deficits, possibly aided by guided work experience. Each procedure takes time, which can be bought by delaying graduation. Family support is crucial to the success of most school and rehabilitation programs, but especially so in the highly charged area of delayed graduation.

Many students with TBI who passed algebra or English literature and graduated from high school on time are now unemployed, living with their families, and unable to manage their own financial affairs. Adolescents with TBI who graduate from high school without becoming aware of their abilities and limitations are at risk for joining adults with TBI who are unemployed.

Summary

Cognitive Retraining

- Offers enhancement of residual cognitive skills
- Is carried out in the classroom
- Uses academic curriculum and daily activities as basis

Common Deficits

- Impaired cognition
- Impaired auditory discrimination
- Restricted visual fields
- Inability to attend to task
- Impaired memory
- Inability to follow a sequence of directions
- Impaired expressive and receptive language capacities
- Increased impulsivity
- Decreased problem-solving ability
- Slowed information processing rate
- Impaired fine- and/or gross-motor skills

- Decreased or absent motivation
- Ineffective strategy choices

Help for Teacher Frustration

- Learn about TBI
- Know the student's relative strengths and weaknesses
- Do not equate physical recovery with cognitive recovery
- Do not be misled by spontaneous reappearance of "islands" of skills
- Be willing to clarify behavioral and instructional expectations often
- Remove or modify environmental behavior triggers
- Assume increased decision-making responsibility for a student with impaired reasoning and judgment

10

Families of Children and Adolescents with Traumatic Brain Injury

Families whose children have sustained TBIs, particularly the recently injured, differ substantially from families whose children have other special education requirements. True, both groups have had to plan for children with special needs. However, the recent experiences of a child's injury and subsequent rehabilitation have profound effects on the family unit and the emotions of its members. Such emotional reactions may make the interchanges between family and school difficult as both plan for the student's program. Although not all families experience the emotional reactions described below, they do frequently occur (Williams & Kay, 1991). Therefore, it is helpful for educators to understand what families have recently experienced and some of the emotional reactions that may color how they perceive school efforts.

Emotional Reactions of the Family

When the family returns their child to school, they have recently been through extremely stressful experiences. During this time, they may

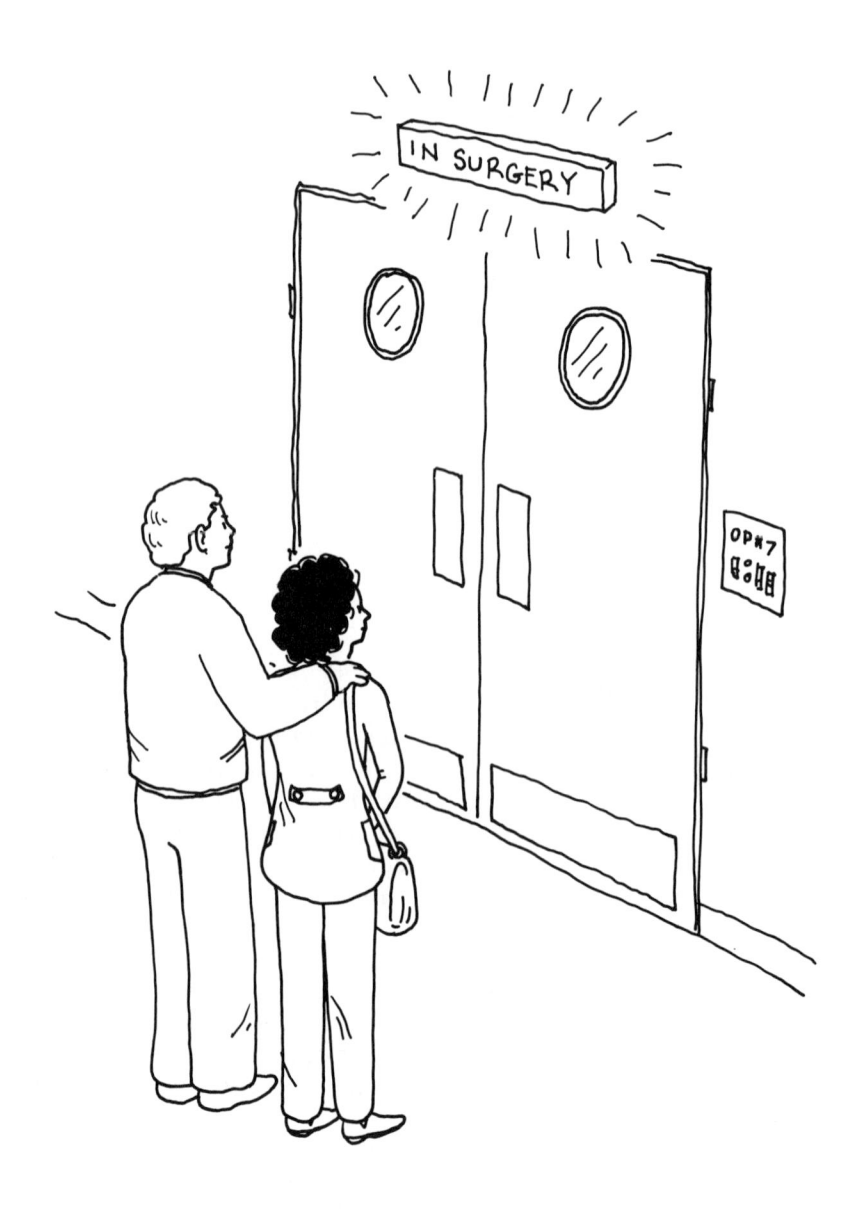

not have taken care of themselves, with long vigils in the hospital disrupting personal routines such as eating and rest.

Family members' first reactions to the trauma are usually *shock* and *disbelief*. Their emotions are intensified by the dramatic surroundings of the accident, trauma care, and, perhaps, surgery. They are fearful for the child's life and uncertain about long-term outcome. For the first time, they may feel their lack of control over their child's life or death. In addition, when they return the child to school, they may be fearful that the school will not understand or be able to provide for the child.

Families also experience *anger* at the injustice of the injury and may direct their anger at persons or events they perceive as responsible for the injury. For example, a parent may express anger at the driver of the car that hit the child, or the spouse who did not supervise, or the medical staff who were not compassionate enough. Anger is commonly directed toward the school if it appears that educators are not doing enough to speed recovery.

Sorrow over the child's pain and need for medical procedures is common, along with *grief* over the loss of the child as he or she was before the accident. Grief is compounded if other family members were injured or killed in the same accident. Family members will experience *depression* that will continue to resurface for many years. As they come to fully appreciate the extent of the resulting disabilities, their depression may intensify.

Family members often experience a certain amount of *guilt*, whether or not any one of them was responsible for the injury. Thus, parents often think, "If only I had . . . , this would not have happened."

Although families differ in their coping styles, even strong families experience the range of emotions outlined here. The changing nature of family reactions following the injury is not a one-way process; emotional reactions will wax and wane. Specific events will trigger the return of reactions that were dominant earlier.

The issues of parental denial and acceptance following a trauma to or illness in their child have received a great deal of attention. *Denial* is a common and lingering response of family members, especially when the child has made enough early progress to negate previous predictions. Such denial is reinforced when a child lives who was expected to die. If parents are told that the child may not regain motor function and if the child indeed does, again disbelief of professionals is reinforced. Denial, as an inability to view the child and the child's potential in the same way as professionals, is not always negative. Rather, it is an important part of the adjustment process as it allows families to continue with lengthy rehabilitation and gives them time to gradually recognize the facts about the injury.

Acceptance of the implications of the TBI means that the family has arrived at a realistic view of the child's disabilities and intact skills, along with realistic expectations for the child's behavior. At this point, the family members accept the changed child. For some, acceptance may come only after a long time; for others, it may never occur.

Sources of Family Distress

If educators are aware of the difficult situations that families face, they will be better able to help families through the process of developing the best possible educational plan.

Lack of Information

It is difficult for families to gain access to factual information about TBI and their children's condition. While the child is in the hospital, the family must deal with sometimes baffling medical terminology and information. As the child progresses, the family finds that it cannot get clear information about long-term expectations for the child. Medical and rehabilitation staff often do not make long-range predictions because they may not feel sufficiently trained or comfortable, they may not have enough information, or they may think that the family is not emotionally ready for negative predictions.

Very little information is available for families about TBI in children. Furthermore, most parents are too tired and distracted to take in much by reading about TBI during the early stages of the child's rehabilitation. When parents receive or assimilate only fragmentary information, they may assemble their own conclusions about their child and the child's prognosis. For example, parents may misinterpret glowing reports about the child's physical recovery as indication of total, including cognitive, recovery. This, in turn, may lead families to reject recommendations for additional therapy or special education services.

Uncertain Outcome

From the time of the trauma, the family is dealing with uncertainty. Initially, parents may not know if their child will live. Even after the child is medically stable, there is uncertainty about what handicaps may be present and whether the child will require long-term inpatient care. When it is time for school reentry, parents are not certain how to approach the school and whether there will be an appropriate program for the child.

Financial Stresses

The TBI itself and subsequent lengthy rehabilitation are financially devastating to most families. Even with insurance, many rehabilitation procedures are not covered, and lifetime caps on spending may lead families to save benefits for possible future needs. Furthermore, family income may be reduced as one member stops working to be with or care for the injured child.

Disruption of Family Life and Roles

Family members' roles may be altered by the injury. A parent who has remained in the background may now have to be the one to carry out all communication with professionals. Siblings may be assigned responsibilities prematurely. Such role changes may lead to conflicts among family members, making marital discord and problems among siblings common.

Behavior Problems

If the child with TBI exhibits serious personality changes or residual behavior problems, the need for the family to learn new management skills comes at a time when the members are physically and emotionally exhausted. It is not unusual for a child to be sent home exhibiting aggressive outbursts to be cared for by a mother who is physically smaller than her child.

Reactions of Siblings

Other children in the family are significantly affected by the injury. Younger children, in particular, may not understand what happened to their brother or sister, and whether he or she will live. Siblings will feel the same emotions of guilt, anger, grief, loss, and even denial as their parents. In addition, they may erroneously feel responsible for the injury. Not only may their responsibilities increase while parents take on the care of the injured child, but siblings may also feel a marked reduction in parental attention during this time, sometimes to the point of neglect.

Siblings may have had to deal with questions from peers and teachers in school. They may be ashamed of the injured child's disabilities, and feel that their own standing with peers may be affected. Parents who are sensitive to the reactions of the injured child's siblings and who try to alleviate them are faced with another major challenge at a time when they are already pressed for energy and time.

Dealing with the Special Education System

When the child's postinjury deficits suggest the need for special education services, families may encounter the special education network and procedures for the first time. This experience may prove difficult and contribute to a family's emotional distress. Some families view special education as something for children who are "handicapped" or "retarded." If they feel that their child is close to total recovery, they see no need to involve special education. The negation of their child's special needs occasionally takes extreme forms. For example, a family may reject the school's offer to transport a child with reduced stamina if it is by the special education bus.

When planning school reentry, many families have become accustomed to the medical routines, which they accept with little discussion. They are eager to get on with their child's education and may impatiently view special education procedures, such as evaluations, staffing, and planning, as foot dragging on the part of the school. Often, therefore, this process intensifies parents' already high level of frustration and anger.

During assessment and interpretation of school evaluations, families may confront the reality of their child's cognitive sequelae for the first time. By presenting the child's deficits and their real world implications, the findings may call back the family's guilt and sorrow and provoke protective reactions in which the family discards the school's findings.

Thus, families will bring to the reentry planning a number of understandable emotions, which may impede their ability to easily participate in the process. Additionally, parents often possess little information about TBI and what schools can do and they have little experience with their changed child. They have limited ability to effectively advocate for their child. Educators need to understand what families are experiencing and the factors that are contributing to their anguish, and may need to make a greater than usual effort to engage the family in the educational planning.

How Schools Can Work with Families of Children with TBI

A number of measures can be taken to facilitate and enhance the relationships between families and the school to ensure the best possible educational program for the child with TBI. These include the following:

• *Provide information.* As educators become knowledgeable about TBI, they can act as information resources for families. As they become familiar with the child's learning characteristics, they are in a better position than most professionals to help parents understand how the child learns and what can be expected in the future.

• *Provide parents an opportunity to view the child realistically.* The school is the best setting in which to observe the impact of cognitive or behavioral residuals of the injury. At school, educators and the child begin to face what the new learning pattern will be. When provided the chance to observe and participate, parents can become a part of this unfolding understanding about the child. Such involvement will help them accept the child's limitations and strengths.

• *Share strategies with parents.* After working with the child, teachers will discover certain methods that are successful for managing behavior, for helping the child at word finding and remembering strings of information, and for keeping the child on task. These methods should regularly be shared with families who, in turn, may have ideas for the school. Encourage parents to participate in their child's education and make them feel that their opinions and observations are valuable.

• *Avoid overreacting to parental criticism.* Educators need to recognize that the family's stress and anger are expressed in many ways. Understanding some of the origins of family reactions and perhaps illogical negative responses to the school will help educators deal reasonably with the families and direct them toward productive avenues.

• *Encourage use of community resources.* Families can be directed toward head injury support groups, where they can meet with others who share similar experiences. The National Head Injury Foundation and affiliated state organizations can assist families in locating a nearby support group.

A family may require respite services, particularly if the child was severely injured and continues to require a great deal of attention and care. This challenge may leave parents with little time for themselves, or a family emergency may require that someone else care for the child for a period. On its own, a family may not be able to find someone who is able to care for the child. School personnel may assist families by directing them to social service agencies or disability support groups who can make a referral to respite care services.

• *Provide help for siblings.* Schools can often provide support and counseling for the injured child's school-age siblings. Be sure their teachers are aware of the changed home situation so they can deal with these students appropriately and be alert to difficulties.

Summary

Family Reactions to a Child's TBI

- Shock and disbelief
- Anger
- Sorrow/depression
- Denial
- Acceptance

Contributors to Family Distress

- Limited information
- Uncertain outcome
- Financial burden
- Disrupted family life
- Siblings' reactions
- Behavior problems
- Dealing with the school system

11

Summary and Implications for Future Directions

Recent legislation establishing a special education category for traumatic brain injury (PL 101-476) is encouraging educators to learn more about TBI. Such legislation was needed because of the significant number of children struggling in school with the residuals of head injury. Prior to this time, no specific definition, reporting method, and manner of documentation were available to identify, study, or accurately track this population. The recognition of TBI as a distinct category will help educators determine the needs of these students and devise appropriate programs for them.

Too often, educators have been ill informed and untrained in TBI. As a result, students with TBI have been classified as mentally retarded, behavior disordered, or learning disabled.

Effects of TBI

Traumatic brain injuries can have profound effects on a child's developing brain. Unpredictable learning and behavior patterns may

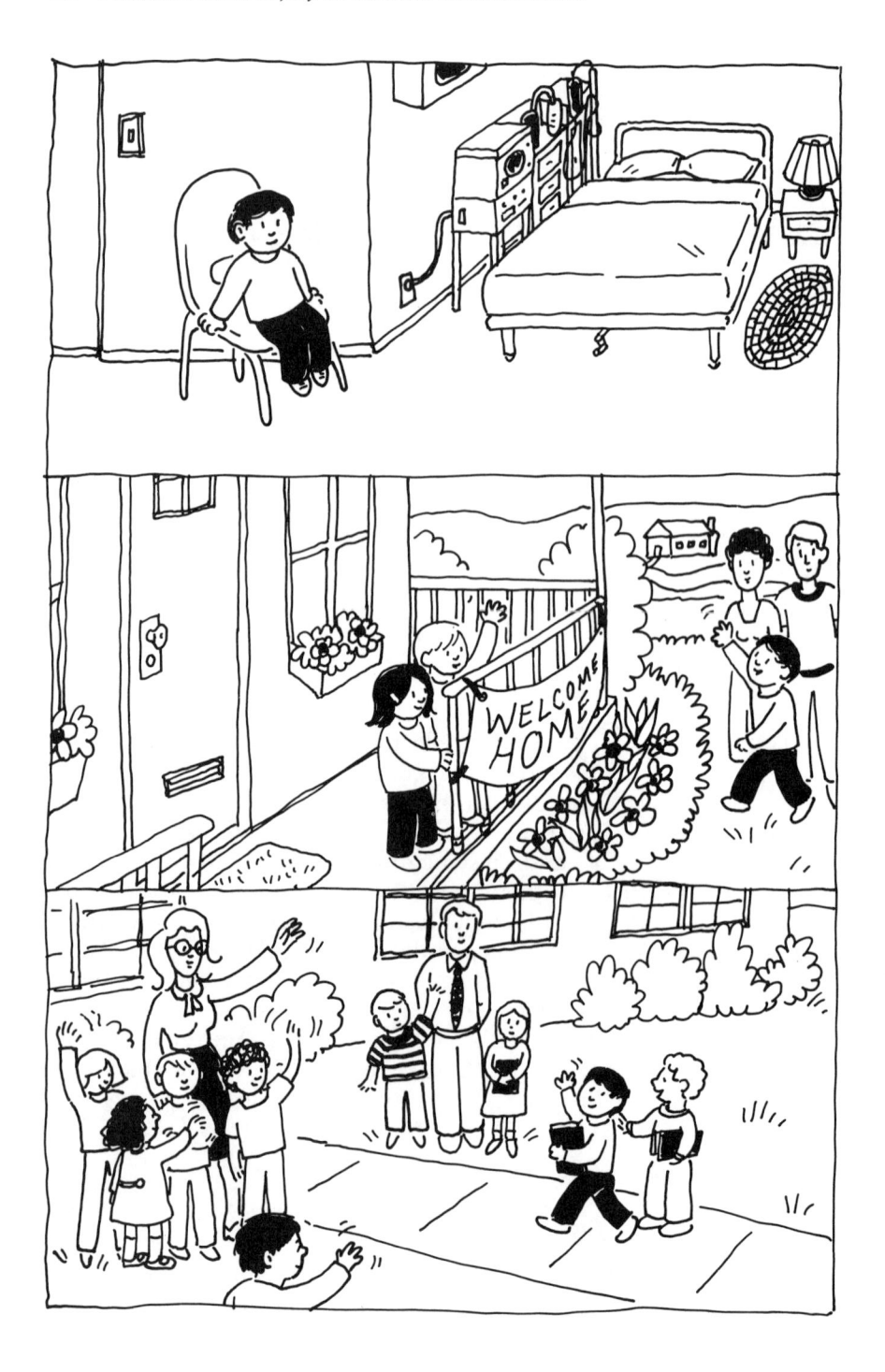

92 *Traumatic Brain Injury in Children and Adolescents*

emerge subsequent to an injury. Rate of development and ultimate level of achievement may be altered. Skills not mastered before an injury may never emerge intact.

Infants, toddlers, and preschoolers with TBI are at greater risk for later learning and behavioral impairments than older children. The commonly held assumption that the brains of younger children are more plastic and will recover more readily and completely is incorrect. Knowledgeable preschool screening teams will ask parents if children have experienced head injuries prior to school entry. It is important to query parents directly because they may consider a TBI at age 2 insignificant 3 years later when it is time for kindergarten, and may not report it. If educators are informed early, they can be alert to children's special needs.

Even if recovery is proclaimed "complete" by physicians, children may return to school following a moderate to severe TBI with a range of deficits in their physical and sensory conditions, cognition, memory, attention, and language. They may have problem-solving and mental processing difficulties.

Amid these deficits, children may display islands of preserved skills, which is sometimes referred to as the "Swiss cheese effect." These skills may mislead educators into thinking that the children are more intact than is the case, and thus to hold unrealistically high expectations. Also, despite the cognitive deficits, children with TBI may still score within the average range on individual IQ and achievement measures. This not only compounds the problem of unrealistic expectations, but has often precluded their receiving needed special education services.

Children with TBI may exhibit a range of problematic or inappropriate behavior. They may say things that are offensive, provocative, or tangential to the topic, or ask questions that cause others discomfort. This behavior following a TBI may so annoy peers that the child who was physically isolated from them for so long now becomes socially isolated.

Reentry to School

The business of childhood is learning. This is emphatically true for children and adolescents following TBI. The school is *the* best place for the relearning necessary after TBI. The structure, commitment to learning, and ordered curriculum available in school are vital for recovery and retraining of students after TBI. Thus, schools are a necessary part of the continuum of services these children require.

The manner in which educators handle the transition from rehabilitation to education is significant, not only for the students' subsequent learning, but for their long-term psychosocial well being. An effective reentry requires a number of features: (a) early, reciprocal communication between medical and educational professionals; (b) the ability of the school to gather, interpret, and translate information about the student's injuries, subsequent improvement course, and residual deficits; (c) procedures, backed by policy, for comprehensive assessment and planning *before* the student returns to school; (d) flexibility to design special programs fitting the student's cognitive, behavioral, and health needs; and (e) a clear mechanism for monitoring and revising the program as needed. Additionally, successful reentry requires that all school personnel working with the student be trained in TBI.

Such reentry planning has been carried out successfully in many schools, for many students with TBI. However, unless school districts have a designated plan to carry out the planning, the re-entry process may be haphazard, or not planned at all. Experience is showing that a key to successful reentry planning and program monitoring lies in having a designated person or team within the school to initiate, coordinate, and evaluate this step-by-step process. We have termed this professional the *case manager*. Although the title is unimportant, the roles are vital for the success of the reentry plan.

Teaching the Student with TBI

The residual deficits of students with TBI must be taken into account in developing appropriate educational programs. Their unique cognitive deficits require cognitive retraining or rehabilitation, which should utilize an academic curriculum appropriate to the student's level of functioning and range of deficits and strengths. Furthermore, the student's specific deficits (e.g., memory or attention problems) will require techniques to help the student compensate for the impaired functioning. Because students with TBI differ from those special education students with developmental disorders, the curricula for those with learning disabilities or mental retardation are neither designed nor appropriate for students with TBI.

The student's physical deficits following TBI may require modifications in scheduling and adaptations in the classroom environment and materials. Provisions for dealing with behavioral problems also need to be in place.

Emerging Issues

Financial Issues

School administrators are not clear where rehabilitation ends and education begins. Therapies provided during rehabilitation are financed by the family or third-party providers; those therapies that are educationally significant are financed by the school. Fiscal responsibilities blur when a student is simultaneously on homebound instruction (at the school's expense) while receiving outpatient rehabilitation therapies (at the family's expense). For now, schools tend to assume financial responsibility for therapies upon the student's actual school reentry.

Training Issues

Passage of PL 101-476 means that all school personnel will need training to become knowledgeable about TBI. Inservice training will be needed for special and regular education teachers, school psychologists, counselors, and social workers. Teacher training institutions may soon offer instruction about TBI. Issues related to certification or recertification may be forthcoming.

Educational Research Issues

Currently, there is little research to point to the soundest procedures for educating students with TBI. We do not know which school reentry procedures are best. We need a clear understanding of the relationship between cognitive abilities and academic achievement after a head injury. We also need to identify the best teaching techniques.

We have little data about which interventions are most effective for reducing emotional and behavioral deficits following TBI. We should know which interventions have greater potential and which ones to avoid (Lehr, 1990).

We have not verified the best ways to assess the range of cognitive effects of a TBI. Tests in the Halstead–Reitan batteries are sensitive to cognitive deficits, but need updating in light of developments in the cognitive and neurological sciences (Bigler, 1990). We know that traditional one-to-one assessment procedures do not reveal the range or depth of students' deficits following TBI. We may need to develop more functional assessment procedures to learn about students in other environments.

Prevention

Because there is no cure for traumatic injuries to the brain, prevention is the only way to avoid their effects. Several state head injury associations and some hospitals are developing programs to boost prevention awareness. Schools are welcoming these programs as another way to educate students about protecting their health and abilities.

APPENDIX A
Bibliography

Begali, V. (1987). *Head injury in children and adolescents: A resource and review for school and allied health professionals.* Brandon, VT: Clinical Psychology.
This paper-bound book includes medical, physiological, rehabilitative, neuropsychological, and behavioral dimensions of traumatic head injury. Its multidisciplinary view is educationally relevant and provides practical information to individualize instruction and capitalize on potential for recovery of students with TBI. It explains ways of using school and community reintegration as extensions of an ongoing rehabilitation process.

Bigler, E. D. (Ed.). (1990). *Traumatic brain injury: Mechanisms of damage, assessment, intervention, and outcomes.* Austin, TX: PRO-ED.
The book is an outgrowth of a series of articles dealing with traumatic brain injury published in the *Journal of Learning Disabilities* in 1987 and 1988. The articles are arranged into sections covering pathologic consequences of injury, assessment issues, intervention issues, and outcome issues. It is a comprehensive source of information on TBI in children and adults. George Prigatano, Linda Ewing-Cobbs, Felicia Goldstein, Harvey Levin, Thomas Marquardt, and Cathy Telzrow are among the contributors to the volume.

Lehr, E. (1990). *Psychological management of traumatic brain injuries in children and adolescents.* Rockville, MD: Aspen.
This book represents research and clinical findings covering head injury rehabilitation from the acute care setting to the return to home and school. It is a resource for physicians, educators, allied health professionals, psychologists, neuropsychologists, insurers, case managers, and parents. It provides insight into the long-term impact of childhood head trauma and gives special emphasis to the behavioral and psychosocial aspects of head injury.

National Head Injury Foundation Task Force on Special Education. (1989). *An educator's manual: What educators need to know about students with traumatic brain injury.* Southborough, MA: NHIF.
This book is a looseleaf-bound volume that discusses educational issues for students with TBI, elements of brain anatomy, assessment and intervention, social and behavioral aspects, and creating a workable education program.

Rosen, C., & Gerring, J. (1986). *Head trauma: Educational reintegration.* San Diego: College-Hill.

This 150-page paper-bound book addresses major problems associated with education for students with traumatic brain injuries. The authors discuss problems and make recommendations for educational management based on their observation and experience as members of a pediatric rehabilitation team in a hospital setting.

Rourke, B. P., Bakker, D. J., Fisk, J. L., & Strang, J. D. (1983). *Child neuropsychology: An introduction to theory, research and clinical practice.* New York: Guilford.

This book provides information on the development and structure of the brain, representation of major functions in the hemispheres, and the brain's capacity to recover after injury. It then addresses the concepts and procedures of neuropsychological assessment of children. It presents in detail the use of neuropsychological data to develop a remedial plan for a child who has sustained a TBI. Over one-third of the book is devoted to case studies of children with a range of neurological disorders. The book is a useful introduction for school psychologists to application of neuropsychological methods of planning for students.

Tyler, J. S. (1990). *Traumatic head injury in school-aged children: A training manual for educational personnel.* Kansas City: University of Kansas Medical Center, Children's Rehabilitation Unit.

This training manual is designed to assist trainers in providing information about head injuries to educators and other professionals who will be working with those children. Included in the training packet is a complete manuscript for a 3-hour training session, diagrams and lists that can be made into slides, handouts, and an 8 minute videotape on school reentry.

Williams, J. M., & Kay, T. (Eds.). (1991). *Head injury: A family matter.* Baltimore: Brookes.

The purpose of this book is to provide the first comprehensive consideration of the impact of head injury on the family system from the perspective of families who have experienced head injury and from professionals who work with those families. Six individuals recount their personal experiences in one section. Another section describes family needs during all phases of service delivery. Another section describes resources and tools to provide the family intervention and support necessary to help the family achieve the optimum level of normalcy after a family member sustains a TBI. The final chapter explains the role and resources of the National Head Injury Foundation.

Ylvisaker, M. (Ed.). (1985). *Head injury rehabilitation: Children and adolescents.* Austin, TX: PRO-ED.

This book will be of interest to all rehabilitation and special education professionals who work with head injured children and adolescents and their families. It provides information on specific treatment techniques and the use of an interdisciplinary approach to pediatric head injury rehabilitation. It is intended to be a practical guide for professionals seeking concrete procedures to effectively treat children with head injuries. It is an in-depth presentation of physical and neurological effects of TBI. It provides extensive programming guidelines for patients in the acute recovery phase; thus, it has information for educators working with severely impaired children.

APPENDIX B
Physical Facilities and Planning Checklist for Schools

Classroom and Halls

____ Are floors of nonslip material?

____ Are water fountains located on each floor?

Does the student:

____ Have to change classes?

____ Have to change levels? (Specify appropriate options—elevator, ramps, stairs with handrails.)

____ Need to be dismissed early to avoid hall traffic?

____ Participate in recess?

____ Need a rest period at school? (Specify length and location.)

____ Carry and manage his or her own books? (Specify person who assists.)

____ Require preferential seating?

Restroom

Does the student:

____ Need assistance in caring for bowel/bladder needs? (Specify appropriate procedures and person who assists.)

____ Have an accessible, private place available for toileting?

____ Have bowel/bladder accidents? (Who assists? Where can extra clothing be kept at school?)

____ Need help with clothing?

____ Need help with physical access to toilet?

____ Need adaptive equipment (e.g., raised toilet seat, grab bars)?

____ Have adequate time for attending to toileting needs?

Cafeteria

Does the student:

____ Have access to the cafeteria?

___ Have a special diet or diet supplement? (Specify diet restrictons. Specify who supplies special foods.)

___ Have ability to manage food tray and eat independently? (Specify person who assists and the needed adaptive eating equipment.)

Gym

Does the student:

___ Have ability to participate in physical education classes?

___ Need adaptive physical education?

___ Need modified sports equipment?

School/Student Awareness

___ Have all appropriate school personnel been briefed or trained regarding the student's medical condition and needs?

___ Have classmates and other peers been informed or trained about medical or behavior needs?

___ Have emergency procedures been defined? Tested?

Does the student:

___ Have an adult advocate at school?

___ Exhibit behavior that might be dangerous to himself/herself or others?

Medical

Does the student:

___ Take medicine at school? (Specify procedures, storage location, person who administers dosage.)

___ Take medication producing side effects?

___ Take medication that affects school performance?

___ Have a history of or current episodes of seizures? (Specify personnel and procedures trained to intervene.)

___ Wear braces or splints, or use assistance for walking?

___ Need humidifying/suction or other equipment for trachea tube care?

Equipment

Does the student:

____ Need other adaptive equipment at school?
    ____ Computer, adaptive hardware, adaptive software
    ____ Typewriter, braillewriter
    ____ Adaptive seating: seat insert, lap tray, standing table
    ____ Augmentative communication: communication board, headstick, mouthstick, other
    ____ Adjustable desktop
    ____ Special paper: wide spaced, raised lines, colored lines
    ____ Special pencils, pen
    ____ Squeeze scissors

Transportation and Parking

____ Are walking surfaces between bus and building of nonslip material?

____ Are curb cuts between bus and building conveniently located?

____ Are there obstacles (manhole covers, ventilation grates) between parking lot and school building?

____ Has transportation facility been informed of schedule, and where to pick up and drop off student?

____ Who accompanies student on bus?

Does the student:

____ Use regular bus service?

____ Use alternative transportation? (Specify alternative.)

____ Need special transportation? (Specify needs—hydraulic chair lift, preferential parking.)

APPENDIX C
Checklist for School Reentry

Things To Do During the Acute Care Phase

Step 1

Rehabilitation medicine consultation with hospital psychology and/or education departments for psychological/ neuropsychological testing and education evaluation and planning assistance.

Step 2

Psychology/education personnel from the hospital review student/ patient's chart, visit patient and family, and check patient and chart daily to determine readiness for appropriate standardized tests and informal assessment.

- ____ Get appropriate consent forms signed by parents
- ____ Exchange information with school
- ____ Include school attendance, achievement, and anecdotal records
- ____ Send hospital records that are relevant to future education planning and programming
- ____ Schedule first testing session if appropriate
- ____ Give family an information packet with materials to inform them of educational needs of students with TBI and support group contacts
- ____ Arrange to videotape student in therapy sessions (tapes may be edited and used later by parents or teachers to facilitate school reentry or document progress)

Step 3

Someone from the hospital should telephone or visit school after parent signs consent forms.

- ____ Discuss student's current condition and estimated time until hospital release
- ____ Discuss arrangements for homebound teaching, if appropriate
- ____ Discuss tentative sequence of events for school reentry, techniques for managing reentry, and resources that may be needed

____ Schedule school representatives' hospital visit with student; also schedule time for them to meet physicians and rehabilitation therapists

____ Inform school personnel of dates, times, and locations of hospital team meetings and planning conferences; make arrangements for their attendance

Step 4

____ Arrange a time and date to conduct inservice for teachers and support personnel; explain considerations in reentry planning

Step 5

Request a written summary for the school

Summary should describe the student's injury, course of treatment and recovery, and recommendations for meeting the student's education needs by modifying the education program and school environment.

Recommendations may include:

____ School-based occupational, physical, or speech therapy

____ Counseling—peer group, academic, behavioral, vocational

____ Planning for emergencies—physical or behavioral problems

____ Medication and dosage schedules

____ Transportation

____ Equipment—wheelchair, oxygen, augmentative communication

____ Adaptive physical education

____ Ways to promote positive self-image and peer interaction

____ Ways to manage apathy, impulsivity, disinhibition, altered judgment

____ Ways to minimize family stress

____ Ways to capitalize on relative academic strengths

____ Ways to minimize or remediate relative academic weaknesses

____ Ways to increase attention, concentration, organization

____ Evaluation/assessment intervals

_____ Timing for team meetings to discuss progress—when to monitor, evaluate, and reprogram

_____ School's liaison with other agencies—vocational rehabilitation, social services, hospital, rehabilitation physicians, community support services

_____ Most appropriate educational service delivery option—resource, self-contained, mainstream, homebound, shortened school day

_____ Inservice program for school personnel or resources for obtaining inservice training

APPENDIX D
Evaluation Summary

Name: Jerry Lane   Date of Hospitalization: 3/20/91-7/7/91
Birth Date: 4/20/74   Case Manager: Beverly Jones, M.S.Ed.
School: Walnut Ridge   Date of Report:7/25/91
Referred by: Dept. Rehabilitation Medicine, Central Medical Center

Accident and Hospital Course

Jerry is a 17-year-old male who was admitted to the Intensive Care Unit of the Central Medical Center following a motor vehicle accident. He sustained multiple fractures and a severe head injury when he was ejected from the vehicle. The CT scan indicated extensive hemorrhaging within the brain, extending into the brain stem. He was comatose for 4 weeks. He was transferred from intensive care to the Rehabilitation Service for therapy on 4/08/91.

During his 3 months in the Rehabilitation Service, Jerry had persistent problems with high blood pressure, which was eventually managed by medication and a salt-free diet. His right tibia fracture was casted and he wore a cervical collar for spine fractures. He progressed rapidly to being upright in a wheelchair and was ambulating for short distances by discharge. He attended classes in the hospital classroom during May.

Visual acuity problems that had been identified by his school prior to the TBI hampered his functioning in the classroom. Repeated efforts to get his prescription for glasses filled were unsuccessful because of lack of parental interest. His acuity problem can be corrected with +3 magnifying glasses. Additionally, he had visual problems that included restricted visual fields and blurring. There are no recommendations for either of these ocular difficulties, which may resolve in 6 months to 1 year.

He was discharged on a prophylactic dose of anticonvulsant medication daily. On discharge, he continued to demonstrate reduced stamina, which suggested that he would not be able to work for more than a half day when he returns to school.

Educational History

School records indicated that Jerry began having learning problems at about the seventh grade. He was evaluated and found eligible for services as a student with learning disabilities. He received resource services in junior high for reading and is presently on a monitor status. He had additional problems of attendance related to his employment in a nursing home. Rather than attending school, he was trying to get a GED independently and pursue a training course for a Licensed Practical Nurse. He is presently behind in credits for graduation and is very concerned about the possibility of having to make up the credits and, consequently, stay in school longer.

Family Situation

Jerry's family consists of his mother, who is employed, and an older sister who lives 600 miles away. No father is in the picture. The problems of family participation during his hospitalization included neglect in signing consent forms for summer school, delays in getting prescription lenses, and infrequent visiting.

Discharge Plan

Jerry's discharge plan included daily attendance in the morning at the Diagnostic Classroom for Learning Problems affiliated with Central Medical Center, and at an adult day care center in the afternoon, where he received occupational, physical, and speech therapy. His school transported him to the diagnostic classroom in the morning and to the adult day care center at noon. This discharge plan was determined partly by the fact that there would be no one at home during the day to help meet his needs. It is anticipated that Jerry will return to school in September; however, a change of school to a more handicapped accessible building is necessary because of his continued physical problems. Additionally, the following recommendations were made by the rehabilitation staff:

1. Follow-up visits in the Departments of Rehabilitation Medicine and Neurology as indicated
2. Follow-up visits in Ophthalmology
3. Audiological evaluation to be performed at school to rule out residual hearing problems following the TBI
4. Self-managed salt-free diet
5. Occupational, physical, and speech therapy to continue after returning to school

Rehabilitation Summary

Jerry received physical, occupational, and speech therapy while in the Rehabilitation Service and attended classes in the hospital classroom during May. Additionally, he had extensive neuropsychological assessment, as well as a diagnostic educational assessment in the diagnostic classroom. The relevant results and recommendations are discussed in the following sections.

Physical Therapy Summary and Recommendations

Jerry has made considerable improvement in physical abilities since the accident. He now ambulates over moderate distances but still uses a wheelchair for longer trips. However, because of poor balance, he falls frequently and requires great effort to get up independently. He continues to have deficits in upper extremity coordination and efficient movements. These problems improve with therapy. The recommendations for physical therapy include the following:

1. Daily physical therapy to continue working on all aspects of gross motor functioning.
2. Improve upper extremity coordination and speed.
3. Continue work on independent ambulation and ability to get up from sitting position.
4. Work on balance.

These skills will allow Jerry to participate more in activities with peers and be more independent in his environment.

Occupational Therapy Summary and Recommendations

Regarding activities of daily living, Jerry continues to require some set-up for grooming and feeding, and opening some containers. He is now dressing but requires some assistance, particularly with fasteners. He is right-hand dominant and is making improvement in fine-motor coordination, particularly in the right upper extremity.

Because of the reported visual acuity problems and possible visual perceptual problems prior to the TBI, he was administered the *Non-Motor Test of Visual Perceptual Skills*. On this test, he functioned with a median perceptual age of 6-6, with a percentile rank of 1%.

The occupational therapy (OT) recommendations include:

1. Direct OT services in the school at least three times a week to enhance upper extremity functioning, particularly on the left.
2. Assistance directed at visual perceptual and cognitive skills.

Speech and Language Summary

Throughout hospitalization and outpatient therapy, Jerry worked on reading, writing legibly with appropriate spelling and punctuation, and following two-step directions. Treatment also focused on auditory recall of information from a three-sentence paragraph to improve his short-term memory. He also worked on sequencing four-step tasks. To develop problem-solving skills, treatment included deriving several solutions to everyday situations. Jerry performed the above tasks with 70–80% accuracy. However, distractibility led to extreme performance variability.

Speech and language recommendations include:

1. Continued language therapy focused on memory and verbal problem-solving skills.
2. An educational rehabilitation program via public school attendance.

Hospital Classroom Summary

Jerry attended the hospital classroom throughout the month of May, receiving approximately 19 hours of instruction. He progressed from requiring all of his work to be read to him and answering questions orally, to reading his own assignments and writing answers on paper. His penmanship and number writing improved, but there was day-to-day variability. Most academic work was at the seventh-grade level, but he could not function independently at that level. He tired easily after an hour of work. His memory difficulty was evident in his requirement to reread material several times in order to answer comprehensive questions. He enjoyed coming to the classroom and interacting with other students. He was almost always positive and ready to get to work. He was interested in regaining his skills so that he could write a report on head injuries.

Neuropsychological Functioning

Jerry was evaluated in the hospital utilizing some measures that had also been used in the school. On the *Wechsler Adult Intelligence Scale–Revised*, he obtained a Verbal IQ of 82, which compared favorably to a previous score of 85. This indicated that he is recalling previously acquired verbal information of a relatively rote nature. This score mirrors his observed verbal interaction skills on a day-to-day basis in the hospital. His Performance IQ of 71 was 30 points lower than pretrauma scores, indicating his problems of visual perception, problem solving, and self-monitoring.

The visual field defects and visual acuity problems complicate his ability to function. His motor problems, particularly reduced efficiency on the left, result in problems of motor output speed. Although he may appear superficially able to enter his previous academic program, he has considerable problems with self-monitoring, problem solving in novel situations, and speeded motor output.

The findings of the neuropsychological evaluation indicate the following recommendations:

1. Provide him additional time to process instructions and to formulate and complete his responses.
2. Allow alternatives to written production whenever possible.
3. Because he has difficulty accurately viewing his abilities, the teachers need to provide clear, but accurate, feedback to him about his performance.

Behavioral and Mental Status

Cognitively, Jerry was quickly orientated to person, place, and time while on the Rehabilitation Service, but never came to fully understand the extent of his injuries. He continues to be easily distracted by irrelevant stimuli, but can be redirected, although with difficulty. He has short-term memory impairment and profited from use of a computer to enhance his immediate recall. In all therapies, he was impulsive, which caused him to rush and make careless errors. His impatience, limited recognition of the seriousness of his injuries, and eagerness to get on with his life without having to go through the necessary steps constitute a major residual problem for him. This makes it necessary to continually review with him the rationale for his therapies.

Academic Status

He was administered the *Woodcock–Johnson Psychoeducational Achievement Test* on July 1, while still an inpatient. He scored in the average achievement range in math, despite his voiced concerns about being unable to remember all of the problem-solving steps. His standard score was comparable to his score from the testing administered the previous year in school.

He scored in the severe deficit range on Reading and Written Language Clusters, indicating significant difficulties with written communication, which will be an additional problem in the classroom.

During his placement in the diagnostic classroom, he made continued recovery of previously acquired information. However, deficits in reading, math, and language continued. His comprehension of written material is on the seventh-grade level. He has specific deficits in vocabulary, sequencing, and understanding causal relationships.

His basic math skills are intact (he understands signs, for example); however, he cannot multiply large numbers because he does not align columns. He has problems with decimals and fractions. He also has considerable trouble with word problems and defining math concepts.

In written language, he has difficulty with punctuation, capitalization, and spelling. In oral language, he has difficulties of slowed speech, word retrieval, tangential speech, and circumlocution.

Based on these findings, the following educational recommendations are made:

1. Provide maximal classroom structure with minimal distractions (e.g., study carrel).

2. Because perceptual problems prevent him from copying material from the board, allow someone to copy the material for him or allow him to dictate into a tape recorder.

3. Allow additional time for producing written material.

4. Plan activities that vary response modes (e.g., perform some math problems with pencil and paper, others with a calculator).

5. Provide sixth- to seventh-grade vocabulary-building activities, perhaps alternating between paper-and-pencil and computer activities.

6. Improve sequencing skills by using activities for which successful completion is contingent upon following a specified sequence (e.g., cooking a favorite food).

7. Monitor him carefully in the classroom to be assured that he is understanding written instructions.

In addition to curricular modifications, the other general suggestions for school include:

1. Jerry will need assistance in getting from class to class because he is new to this high school building and his mobility and balance continue to be impaired.

2. Keep a pair of +3 reading glasses at school. He has lost or broken several pairs and has demonstrated difficulty getting around each day without breaking his glasses.

3. Maintain a duplicate set of books at home to reduce his need to carry them to and from school.

4. Allow him extra time for information processing and task completion.

5. External aids such as lists, diaries, computers, and calculators may assist his recall. He may also be helped by being taught internal strategies, such as mnemonics, acronyms, and sequencing.

6. Because of limited family support, use the school counselor to develop a supportive network for him in school.

Because Jerry continues to improve rapidly, a part of his school entry educational plan should include provision for 30-day monitoring during the first semester.

APPENDIX E
Neuropsychological Report

Name: MJ
Chronological Age: 12-6

Referral and History

M sustained a severe head injury 8 weeks prior to this evaluation. He was struck by a car while riding his bicycle; although the car was moving slowly, he bounced onto the hood, striking his head on the windshield. He sustained right frontal and left temporal lobe contusions, as well as subsequent cerebral edema. He also had a nondepressed right frontal skull fracture. He was unresponsive at the accident, gradually becoming more responsive to lesser stimuli over the first week. Four days following the accident, he opened his eyes intermittently to voice; 9 days later, he was exhibiting some spontaneous eye opening and purposeful movement. Ten days following the accident, he was occasionally awake and intermittently responsive to commands.

Prior to the accident, he was an average student. He was reportedly free of behavioral problems and was characterized as a very likable person.

Procedures

Wechsler Intelligence Scale for Children–Revised (WISC–R)
Halstead–Reitan Neuropsychological Battery for Children
Aphasia Screening Test
Category Test

Results

Sensory Perception. There were no indications of tactile imperception with either hand. He was able to recognize bilateral, simultaneous touch to hand, and hand and face. His performance was one standard deviation below average with each hand on tests for finger agnosia (recognizing which finger was touched with eyes closed), and two standard deviations below on the right for recognition of numbers written on the fingers.

There was no evidence of auditory imperception; however, formal audiological assessment had indicated slight difficulty discriminating words in a noisy background. Although there was no evidence of visual imperception or suppression, he has restricted visual fields. In examining for bilateral visual perception, it was necessary to bring the fingers almost to the corner of his eye on the left and a few inches in on the right. There was no indication of visual neglect. On informal observation, his restricted visual fields are not apparent in the way in which he approaches table-top tasks. Also, he was able to work with stimuli presented at a distance.

Implications. Continued problems of tactile perception reflect the continued underlying neurological problems and his difficulty with performing mental operations. Because of the visual field deficit, it will be important to monitor impact in terms of his safety, such as on the playground and his functioning in the classroom. It will be important to be sure that any impulsivity in approaching tasks does not lead him to overlook any dimensions of the task. Modification of the work field may be necessary, such as providing cues to encourage him to scan all material.

Because he may not accurately perceive words out of context in a noisy environment, it will be important to check on his comprehension.

Motor and Psychomotor Skill. M is right handed and footed. Grip strength is approximately equal bilaterally, although the left appears slightly stronger than the right on informal measures. Psychomotor coordination under timed conditions (WISC–R Coding) was significantly reduced. Performance on the Trails Test, requiring him to rapidly draw lines connecting a series of numbered circles, was reduced. Speed of name writing was slightly below average. Simple motor efficiency as measured by finger tapping is reduced bilaterally. Other measures of motor skill and strength were not attempted because of time. Levels of performance for each hand on the *Tactual Performance Test* (TPT) were from one to two standard deviations above average, and there were no difficulties utilizing a tactile strategy.

Implications. M demonstrates residuals in simple motor and complex psychomotor efficiency. It can be expected that work output will be reduced. Also, slow work rates will interact with his memory deficits. It takes him so long to complete a task that he may forget what he is doing.

Visual-Spatial Organizational Abilities. On the Performance Scales on the WISC-R, he functioned within average limits on all measures of visual analysis and synthesis, and attention to detail. With the exception of the Coding subtest, which was two standard deviations below the mean, all subtests were within average limits, even without making concessions for speed. Level of performance on the Target Test, a measure of immediate memory for visual sequences, was three standard deviations below average, indicating marked difficulty with the recall of visually presented sequences. On the Trails Test, requiring him to search an array of stimuli while rapidly shifting problem-solving sets, he appeared to have problems with motor processing and speed, but not with the visual search component. His drawings on the *Aphasia Screening Test*, as well as his copying of words, were executed slowly. Since the baseline testing a month ago, there has been improvement in maturity and visual spatial detail, although there are still problems with judgment about organization and placement on the page.

Implications. There are no major problems in this area, but his ability to organize and set up a task is impaired such that he may need support and guidance in the classroom.

Rote Memory. His scores on the Information and Digit subtests of the WISC-R were significantly reduced. Additionally, his ability to recall sentences was one standard deviation below average, and his ability to perform an auditory closure task was significantly impaired by his memory difficulty. His memory for the figures on the TPT was significantly impaired. It was noted during the entire evaluation that if he was distracted from a task, he could not go back and complete it because he lost his train of thought. Memory difficulties are apparent on rote material, as well as on tasks requiring effortful processing, such as the Target Test, and in incidental memory, as on memory for figure location on the TPT.

Implications. It will be important to repeat instructions and use short informational bits. Supplemental visual stimuli should be used whenever possible. Problems that compound his memory difficulty are his slow mental processing and his reduced motor speed, which encourage forgetting before the task is completed. He will require much greater than normal amounts of time to complete tasks.

Speech and Language Characteristics. M's appreciation of basic auditory information without reliance on semantic features is within normal limits. He was adequate on his performance on the *Seashore Rhythm Test*, requiring him to identify similarities or differences in two nonlinguistic sound patterns. He also was within normal limits on the *Speech Sound Perception Test*, requiring him to identify the nonsense word from a group of three words presented.

Misspellings continue on the *Aphasia Screening Test* and are particularly pronounced on oral spelling. He does not yet review work adequately to pick up his misspellings. His functioning on the *Auditory Closure Test* was two standard deviations below average. On the verbal fluency test, requiring generation of word lists on the basis of phonemic cuing, his performance was significantly impaired (-3 standard deviations), which indicates a tendency to have greater difficulty on high-demand tasks. Performance on verbal tasks that require some degree of verbal processing was better than on those of a more rote nature. Oral motor praxis, measured by imitation of multisyllabic words, was within average limits.

His conversations during the evaluation were marked by a reliance on pat, stereotypic phrases, and some perseveration. Although there has been improvement in the aphasic symptoms of naming and word finding, these continue to be present. He does now, however, self-correct when he makes a gross error of naming. Ability to use speech to guide his motor or constructional performance is improving.

Implications. Context and meaning may aid M's functioning on verbal tasks. On confrontational verbal tasks, if he blocks because of word finding difficulty, it will not be helpful if he is pressured to try to work his way out of the situation. Rather, he should be supplied with cues or allowed to move on to the next task.

Nonverbal Problem Solving, Concept Formation. His performance on the *Category Test*, a measure of hypothesis generation and use of feedback, was significantly below average. If he could immediately identify the rule directing the subtest, he could continue to use this principle if provided with positive feedback. However, if his initial hypothesis was incorrect, he could not use feedback to help him shift to a new strategy. His difficulty seems to be with using informational feedback to change performance, rather than with problem solving under novel circumstances, because he did very well on the TPT, a novel task. He showed positive transfer of training on the TPT, with performance improving over the three trials. Thus, it seems that the perseveration and difficulty with flexible and adaptive applications of problem-solving strategies are interfering with his ability to function in complex situations.

Because M gets stuck on one response in complex tasks, he will require prompting to help him select and consider alternative responses.

Impressions. There has been continued improvement in M's functioning over the past several weeks. His ability to tap previously acquired information is returning. His ability to problem solve with relatively straightforward visual spatial tasks, such as those measured by the WISC–R Performance subtests, is now within average limits. However, multiple deficits continue to be present. First, he is significantly handicapped when he must process at a purely mental level without benefit of visual cues. He also rapidly loses information that he is to be manipulating. He is doing a bit better in drawing from previously stored information than in coding and committing to memory new information.

Problems of psychomotor speed and efficiency, as well as some problems with judgment about visual–spatial organization continue. He processes information slowly, partly because he cannot keep in mind all of the necessary pieces. Additionally, there are some continued difficulties with executive functions, such as attention and higher level problem solving. A major difficulty M is showing at the present time is his inability to focus his attention in the presence of any distractions. If he is momentarily distracted and returns to a task, he cannot retrieve the informational bits that he was using to problem solve.

Recommendations

It would be erroneous to look only at the return of M's previously acquired skills and plan his educational program to build on that. He has continued deficits with foundation skills of attention, concentration, and memory. Continued language difficulties of word finding and verbal storage of new information and difficulties with higher level problem solving will dictate concessions in the educational setting. Because of his distractibility, it will be important for him to receive his education in a relatively stimulus-free environment. He is not ready to work beyond the one-to-one level in an instructional setting.

The strategy for his programming should not be on building new information at a grade-expected pace. Rather, it should be to continue to work on impaired cognitive areas using academic material to assist in his cognitive retraining.

Because he continues to change rapidly, all educational programming should be reviewed every 30 days. Additionally, a comprehensive neuropsychological reevaluation should be scheduled at the end of the semester.

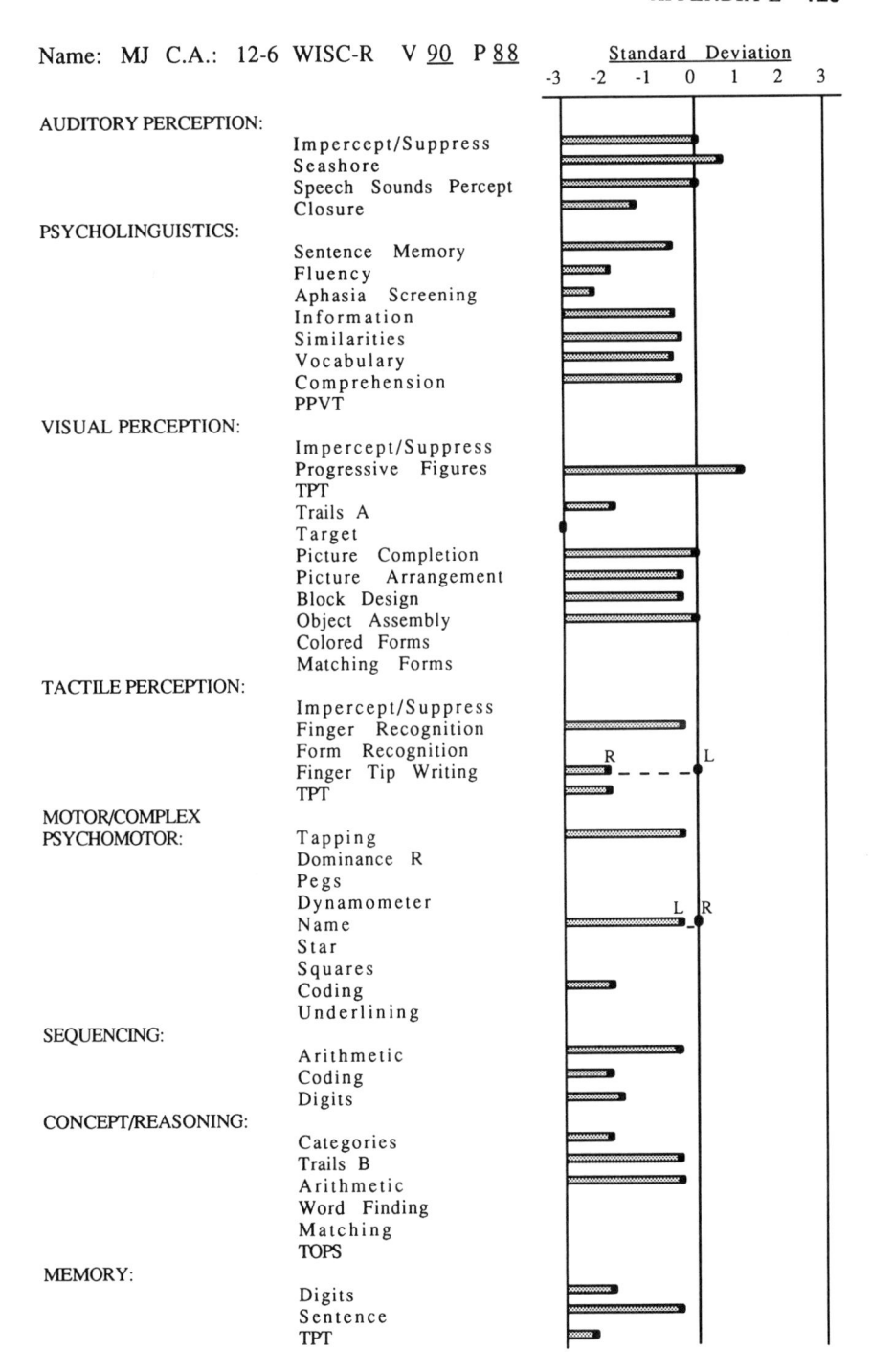

APPENDIX E **123**

Name: MJ C.A.: 12-6 WISC-R V 90 P 88   Standard Deviation
                                          -3 -2 -1 0 1 2 3

AUDITORY PERCEPTION:
    Impercept/Suppress
    Seashore
    Speech Sounds Percept
    Closure

PSYCHOLINGUISTICS:
    Sentence Memory
    Fluency
    Aphasia Screening
    Information
    Similarities
    Vocabulary
    Comprehension
    PPVT

VISUAL PERCEPTION:
    Impercept/Suppress
    Progressive Figures
    TPT
    Trails A
    Target
    Picture Completion
    Picture Arrangement
    Block Design
    Object Assembly
    Colored Forms
    Matching Forms

TACTILE PERCEPTION:
    Impercept/Suppress
    Finger Recognition
    Form Recognition
    Finger Tip Writing
    TPT

MOTOR/COMPLEX
PSYCHOMOTOR:
    Tapping
    Dominance R
    Pegs
    Dynamometer
    Name
    Star
    Squares
    Coding
    Underlining

SEQUENCING:
    Arithmetic
    Coding
    Digits

CONCEPT/REASONING:
    Categories
    Trails B
    Arithmetic
    Word Finding
    Matching
    TOPS

MEMORY:
    Digits
    Sentence
    TPT

Glossary

This glossary contains terms used in this text and/or frequently found in TBI literature. Some are noted initially in the text with italic type and briefly defined there, either parenthetically or in context. This glossary is not a comprehensive list of common TBI terms. It is arranged alphabetically rather than by categories.

anoxia—Condition in which the body receives no oxygen.
antihypertensive—Drug or mode of treatment that reduces blood pressure.
aphasia—Loss of power of expressive speech, writing, or signs, or of comprehending spoken or written language.
apraxia—Impairment in ability to perform purposeful acts in the absence of paralysis or partial paralysis.
ataxia—A disturbance in muscular coordination that may result in dysarthric speech, muscle tremors, or impaired balance.
atrophy—A wasting away of an organ or body tissue.
cognition—The process of knowledge or perceiving.
coma—A state of deep or prolonged unconsciousness, usually caused by injury or illness.
concussion—Condition of impaired functioning of the brain as a result of a violent blow or impact.

confabulation—Fabrication of experiences or thoughts.
contra-coup—Rebound effects of a blow or impact.
contusion—Hemorrhage of capillaries resulting in bruising and swelling.
cortex—Outer convoluted surface of brain made up of nerve cells and their connections.
coup—A blow or impact.
depressed skull fracture—Break in a skull bone with a visible indentation.
diplopia—Double vision.
dysarthria—Incoordination of speech-producing apparatus, causing difficulty in producing speech.
edema—swelling.
endotracheal tube—Catheter inserted through nose or mouth to deliver oxygen, control breathing, or prevent foreign material from entering the lungs.
epilepsy—See *posttraumatic epilepsy*.
gastrostomy tube—A tube surgically inserted into the stomach and used for feeding.
Glasgow Coma Scale—Standardized system for assessing degree of conscious impairment and predicting outcome following traumatic brain injury.

Glasgow Coma Scale

Eye opening	
spontaneous	4
to speech	3
to pain	2
none	1

Best motor response	
obeys commands	6
localizes	5
withdraws	4
abnormal flexion	3
extensor response	2
none	1

(continued)

Verbal response
is oriented	5
confused conversation	4
inappropriate words	3
incomprehensible sounds	2
none	1

On this scale, the score is the total of the three categories of response. Maximum score on this scale is 15 and minimum is 3. The most severely injured persons score the lowest.

hemianopsia—Loss of half of the visual field.
hemiparesis—Muscular weakness on one side of the body.
hemiplegia—Paralysis of one side of the body.
herniation—Protrusion of a portion of the brain through an opening or tear in a membrane or other tissue.
hyperphagia—Voracious overeating caused by damage to the hypothalamus or as a result of disinhibition or both.
hyperthermia—Higher than normal body temperature.
hypotonicity—Low muscle tone in the trunk or extremities.
intracranial hematoma—A local swelling within the brain, filled with blood and causing pressure that slows or stops blood flow or clots and may cause infection.
intracranial pressure (ICP)—Exertion of force within the brain by fluid buildup capable of interrupting cerebral blood flow.
intubation—Insertion of a tube through the mouth or nose to provide an airway for oxygen or anesthetic.
nasogastric tube—Tube inserted through the nostril into the stomach for providing nourishment when the patient cannot ingest food by mouth.
perseveration—Response that is repeated over and over whether or not it is appropriate.
posttraumatic amnesia (PTA)—The interval between injury and the point where memory for daily events and orientation to time and place becomes continuous.
posttraumatic epilepsy—Seizure disorder that results from an injury to the brain.
primary effects—Injury to the brain caused by the injury and subsequent rebounding action.

prophylactic—Medication or procedure administered or performed to prevent negative effects.

Rancho Los Amigos Scale—An 8-point scale that quantifies cognitive recovery after a head injury.

Rancho Los Amigos Levels of Cognitive Functioning

I. no response
II. generalized response
III. localized response
IV. confused, agitated
V. confused, inappropriate, nonagitated
VI. confused, inappropriate
VII. automatic, appropriate
VIII. purposeful, appropriate

residual impairments—Long-lasting or permanent effects of a brain injury.

retrograde amnesia—Inability to remember events preceding an injury.

secondary effects—Injuries caused by bleeding or swelling of the brain subsequent to an injury.

sequelae—Consequences or aftereffects of an injury.

shearing—A brain lesion that results from abrupt deceleration in movement; tears in nerve fibers, especially axons, throughout the brain's white matter.

skull fracture—A break in the bony framework of the head that protects the brain.

spasticity—Uncontrolled contractions or spasms of the skeletal muscles.

ventricles—Cavities inside the brain that normally contain cerebrospinal fluid.

References

Annegers, J. F. (1983). The epidemiology of head trauma in children. In K. Shapiro (Ed.), *Pediatric head trauma* (pp. 1–10). Mount Kisco, NY: Futura.

Bigler, E. D. (Ed.). (1990). *Traumatic brain injury: Mechanisms of damage, assessment, intervention, and outcomes* (pp. 416–417). Austin, TX: PRO-ED.

Brooks, N., McKinlay, W., Symington, C., Beattie, A., & Campsie, B. A. (1987). Return to work within the first seven years of severe head injury. *Brain Injury, 1,* 5–19.

Brown, G., Chadwick, O., Shaffer, D., Rutter, M., & Traub, M. (1981). A prospective study of children with head injuries: Psychiatric sequelae. *Psychological Medicine, 11,* 63–78.

Cohen, S., Joyce, C., Rhoades, K., & Welks, D. (1985). Educational programming for head injured students. In M. Ylvisaker (Ed.), *Head injury rehabilitation: Children and adolescents* (pp. 383–411). Austin, TX: PRO-ED.

Ewing-Cobbs, L., Iovino, I., Fletcher, J. M., Miner, M. E., & Levin, H. S. (1991, February). *Academic achievement following traumatic brain injury in children and adolescents.* Paper presented at the 19th Annual Meeting of the International Neuropsychological Society, San Antonio.

Hagan, C., Malkmus, D., & Durham, P. (1979). Levels of cognitive functioning. *Rehabilitation of the head injured adult: Comprehensive physical management.* Downey, CA: Professional Staff Association of Rancho Los Amigos Hospital.

REFERENCES

Hauser, W. A. (1983). Post-traumatic epilepsy in children. In K. Shapiro (Ed.), *Pediatric head trauma* (pp. 271–287). Mount Kisco, NY: Futura.

Individuals with Disabilities Education Act. (1990, October 30). 20 USC. Sec. 1400-1485 as amended by PL 101-476, Title I, Sec. 101, Title IX, Sec. 1901(b) (10)–(20), 104 Stat. 1103–1142.

Klonoff, H., Low, M. D., & Clark, C. (1977). Head injuries in children: A prospective five year follow-up. *Journal of Neurology, Neurosurgery, & Psychiatry, 40*, 1211–1219.

Kraus, F. J. (1987). Epidemiology of head injury. In P. R. Cooper (Ed.), *Head injury* (2nd ed., pp. 1–19). Baltimore: Williams & Wilkins.

Kraus, J. F., & Nourjah, P. (1989). The epidemiology of mild head injury. In H. S. Levin, H. M. Eisenberg, & A. L. Benton (Eds.), *Mild head injury* (pp. 8–22). New York: Oxford University Press.

Lehr, E. (1990). *Psychological management of traumatic brain injuries in children and adolescents* (pp. 235–236). Rockville, MD: Aspen.

Mira, M. (1989, April). *Educational impact of traumatic head injury in school aged children.* Paper presented at 67th Annual Meeting of the Council for Exceptional Children, San Francisco.

National Head Injury Foundation Task Force on Special Education. (1989). *An educator's manual: What educators need to know about students with traumatic brain injury.* Southborough, MA: NHIF.

P.L. 94-142. (1975). U.S. Congressional and Administrative News, 94th Congress, First Session. *Legislative History, 1*, 773–796. St. Paul, MN: West Publishing.

Reitan, R. M. (1969). *Manual for administration of neuropsychological test batteries for adults and children.* Tucson: Author.

Reitan, R. M., & Davison, L. A. (Eds.). (1974). *Clinical neuropsychology: Current status and applications.* Washington, DC: Winston.

Reitan, R. M., & Wolfson, D. (1985). *The Halstead–Reitan neuropsychological test battery: Theory and clinical interpretation.* Tucson: Neuropsychological Press.

Teasdale, G., & Jennette, B. (1974). Assessment of coma and impaired consciousness: A practical scale. *Lancet, 2*, 81–84.

Wiederholt, J. L. (1974). Historical perspectives on the education of the learning disabled. In L. Mann & D. Sabatino (Eds.), *The second review of special education* (pp. 103–152). Philadelphia: JSE Press.

Williams, J. M., & Kay, T. (Eds.). (1991). *Head injury: A family matter.* Baltimore: Brookes.

Yager, J. Y., Johnston, B., & Seshia, S. S. (1990). Coma scales in pediatric practice. *American Journal of Diseases of Children, 144*, 1088–1091.

Index

Abrasion, effect on brain, 14
Abuse-related traumatic brain injury, 6
Academic problems
  as effect of traumatic brain injury, 23–24, 65–66
  programming for, 72, 74–76
Acceptance, 86
Accidents, 6
Acute care treatment phase, 35, 38–39
Adolescents
  overprotection of, 30
  psychosocial effects of traumatic brain injury on, 11, 29–31
  school-related problems of, 30–31
  sexual interests of, 30
  substance abuse and, 31
Affective disturbances, 28

Age
  influence on traumatic brain injury, 10
  psychosocial effects and, 29
Alcohol abuse, 31
Amnesia, 16, 17
Anger, 85
Antihypertensive medication, 16
Apraxia, 17
Assessment
  components of a neuropsychological examination, 61–62
  differences between neuropsychological and other evaluations, 62–63
  implications of neuropsychological deficits for classroom functioning, 65–66
  importance of neuropsychological examination, 60–61
  longitudinal nature of, 59–60
  neuropsychological batteries, 63

131

research issues on, 96
sample evaluation summary, 109–115
sample neuropsychological report, 117–123
understanding neuro-psychological findings, 65
Ataxia, 17
Attention problems
as effect of traumatic brain injury, 21, 66
programming for, 72
Auditory discrimination, programming for, 71

Behavior abnormalities, 17
Behavior/emotional problems
dealing with, 76–77
as effect of traumatic brain injury, 22–23
impact on family, 87
Bibliography, 97–99
Brain
characteristics of an injured brain, 14–15
cortex of, 15
damage to, 13–14
effect of abrasion on, 14
effect of impact on, 13
effect of stretching on, 13
functions of, 1–2
ongoing development of, 9–10
primary damage to, 13–14
secondary damage to, 14
ventricles of, 15

Calendar, school, 52–53
Career/life planning, 28–29, 79–81
Case management, of school reentry, 39, 54–56
Causes, of traumatic brain injury, 6
Checklists
physical facilities and planning checklist for schools, 101–103
school reentry, 105–107

Classmates, 28, 50
Cognitive problems
as effect of traumatic brain injury, 20–21
programming for, 72, 74–76
Cognitive retraining
educator's role in, 70–71
within the school, 69–70
Coma, 15–16
Community colleges, 80
Community resources, 89–90
Community responses, 79
Computers, and cognitive retraining, 71
Concentration difficulties, 21, 66
Concussion, 5
Contra-coup, 13
Contusion, 6
Cortex of brain, 15
Coup, 13

Daily scheduling, 52–53
Denial
of family, 85–86
of injury, 23
Depression, 85
Developmental aspects of traumatic brain injury
age influence on, 10
disruption of social development and, 10–11
ongoing brain development and, 9–10
Directions, programming for, 74
Disbelief, 85
Drug abuse, 31
Dysarthria, 22

Early acute phase of traumatic brain injury, 15–17
Education. *See* Educators; School reentry; Schools; Special education
Education for all Handicapped Children Act, 1

Educators
　dealing with behavior problems, 76–77
　frustration of, 78–79
　importance of, 45
　inservice training for, 46, 47, 49, 56
　programming for specific deficits, 71–76
　reactions to long-term effects of traumatic brain injury, 77–78
　role in cognitive retraining, 70–71
　skills in understanding neuropsychological findings, 65
Effects of traumatic brain injury. *See* Physical effects of traumatic brain injury; Psychosocial effects of traumatic brain injury
Emotional problems. *See* Behavior/emotional problems
Emotional reactions, of families, 83–86
Epilepsy, posttraumatic, 18
Evaluation, of school environment, 51–52. *See also* Assessment

Families
　behavior problems and, 87
　dealing with the special education system, 88–89
　disruption of family life and roles, 27, 87
　emotional reactions of, 83–86
　financial stresses on, 87
　how schools can work with, 89–90
　information for, 56
　lack of information as source of distress for, 86
　reactions of siblings, 27, 87–88, 90
　school reentry and, 49–50
　sources of family distress, 27, 86–89
　uncertain outcome as source of distress for, 86–87

Fatigue, 18, 53
Financial issues, 40–41, 87, 95

Gastrostomy tube feedings, 16
Glasgow Coma Scale, 15–16
Glossary, 125–128
Goals, educational, 44–45

Halstead-Reitan tests, 63, 96
Headaches, 18
Hearing problems
　as effects of traumatic brain injury, 20
　programming for, 71
Hemorrhage, 14
Homebound education, 36, 53
Hospitals
　hospital-to-school transition planning, 47–51
　interactions with schools, 43–44
　school interactions with, 38–39
　treatment for traumatic brain injury, 35
Hypothermia, 16

ICU. *See* Intensive care unit (ICU)
IEP, 53–54
Impact, effect on brain, 13
Impulsivity
　as effect of traumatic brain injury, 23
　programming for, 74
Incidence, of traumatic brain injury, 3, 5
Independence, problems of, 28, 30
Individuals with Disabilities Education Act, 1
Inservice education. *See* Training
Intellectual problems
　as effect of traumatic brain injury, 21
　programming for, 74–75
Intensive care unit (ICU), 35
Interaction of problems resulting from traumatic brain injury, 24–25

Intracranial hematoma, 6
Intracranial pressure, 16
IQ scores, 21, 62, 63

Language problems
  as effect of traumatic brain injury, 21–22
  programming for, 74
Learning disabilities, compared with traumatic brain injury, 2, 94
Legislation, 1, 43, 91, 95
Life planning, 79–81
Longitudinal nature, of assessment, 59–60

Mathematics skills, 23–24
Medical problems, 16–17
Medication, for behavioral/emotional problems, 23
Meetings, 55
Memory impairment
  as effect of traumatic brain injury, 17, 20–21, 66
  programming for, 72
Mild brain injuries, 5
Moderate brain injuries, 5
Motivation, programming for, 75
Motor problems
  as effect of traumatic brain injury, 17
  programming for, 75
Motor vehicle accidents, 6

Nasogastric tube feedings, 16
Neuropathology, of traumatic brain injury, 13–14
Neuropsychological examination
  battery of tests used in, 63
  compared with other evaluations, 62–63
  components of, 61–62
  importance of, 60–61
  sample evaluation summary of, 109–115
  sample neuropsychological report, 117–123
  understanding findings of, 65

Outpatient rehabilitation, 36
Overactivity, 23
Overprotection, 30

Parents. *See* Families
Peer relationships, 28, 50
Physical effects of traumatic brain injury
  academic effects, 23–24
  behavior abnormalities, 17
  behavioral/emotional effects, 22–23
  characteristics of an injured brain, 14–15
  cognitive effects, 20–21
  coma, 15–16
  initial effects of injury, 15–17
  interaction of problems, 24–25
  language effects, 21–22
  medical problems, 16–17
  memory disorders, 17
  motor problems, 17
  neuropathology of traumatic brain injury, 13–14
  persisting effects, 18–24
  persisting physical effects, 18, 20
  posttraumatic amnesia, 16
  sensory effects, 20
Physical facilities and planning checklist for schools, 101–103
Postacute care, 36
Posttraumatic amnesia (PTA), 16
Posttraumatic epilepsy, 18
Prevention, 96
Primary damage, to brain, 14
Problem solving, programming for, 74
Programming for students with traumatic brain injury
  auditory discrimination, 71
  cognitive retraining within the school, 69–70

dealing with behavior problems, 76–77
educator's role in cognitive retraining, 70–71
for expressive language, 74
for following directions, 72
general modifications for assignments, 75–76
for impulsiveness, 74
for lack of effective strategies, 75
for lack of motivation, 75
for maintaining attention, 72
for memory, 72
for motor skills, 75
for problem solving, 74
for receptive language, 74
research issues on, 95
for restricted visual field, 72
for slow processing, 74–75
sources of teacher frustration, 78–79
for specific deficits, 71–76
teacher reactions to long-term effects of traumatic brain injury, 77–78
Psychosocial effects of traumatic brain injury on adolescents, 29–31
affective disturbances, 28
age considerations, 29
career goals and, 28–29
disorders in family relationships, 27
disruption of social development, 10–11
peer relationships, 28
problems of independence, 28
school's role in, 31–32
PTA. *See* Posttraumatic amnesia (PTA)

Rancho Los Amigos Scale, 16
Reading ability, 24
Recovery. *See* Treatment for traumatic brain injury
Reentry to school. *See* School reentry

Rehabilitation, 36, 39, 40–41
Rehabilitation professionals, 43–44
Research issues, 95–96
Retrograde amnesia, 17
Risk factors, for traumatic brain injury, 6–7

Safety, in schools, 45
Scheduling, daily, 52–53
School calendar, 52–53
School case managers
as communication link, 39, 54
as information resource for family and school, 56
as inservice coordinator, 56
as meeting convener and moderator, 55
as translator, 55
School reentry
barriers impeding successful school reintegration, 46–47
case management of, 54–56
checklist for, 105–107
classmates' preparation for, 50
critical elements that should be in place in schools, 45–46, 101–103
educational goals for students with traumatic brain injury, 44–45
establishing communication between rehabilitation professionals and schools, 43–44
evaluation and modification of the school environment, 51–52
family's reactions to, 88–89
framework for developing an educational plan following traumatic brain injury, 43
homebound education and, 36
hospital-to-school transition planning, 47–51
IEP planning, 53–54
implications of neuropsychological deficits on, 65–66, 94–95
parents' preparation for, 49–50
planning for, 43–56, 93–94

preparation of student with traumatic brain injury for, 50–51
readiness assessment for, 38
school calendar and daily scheduling, 52–53
staff's importance in, 45, 46, 47, 49
variables associated with, 38
Schools. *See also* Special education
and adolescent traumatic brain injury, 30–31
and financing the rehabilitation/recovery program, 40–41
cognitive retraining and, 69–70
communication with rehabilitation professionals, 43–44
dealing with behavior problems, 76–77
educational research issues on, 95–96
educator's role in cognitive retraining, 70–71
evaluation and modification of the school environment, 51–52
family's dealings with special education, 88–89
homebound education and, 36
implications of neuropsychological deficits for classroom functioning, 65–66
information for, 56
interactions with families, 89–90
interactions with hospitals, 38–39, 43–44
physical facilities and planning checklist for, 101–103
programming for specific deficits, 71–76
programming for students with traumatic brain injury, 69–81, 94–95
role in career/life planning, 79–81
role in psychosocial outcome, 31–32
safety in, 45
skills in understanding neuropsychological findings, 65
sources of teacher frustration, 78–79
staff of, 45, 46, 47, 49
teacher reactions to long-term effects of traumatic brain injury, 77–78
Secondary damage, to brain, 14
Seizures, 18
Sensory problems
as effects of traumatic brain injury, 20
programming for, 71, 72
Severe brain injuries, 6
Severity, of traumatic brain injury, 5–6
Sexuality, 30
Shock, 85
Siblings, 27, 87–88, 90
Slow processing, programming for, 74–75
Social development, disruption of, 10–11. *See also* Psychosocial effects of traumatic brain injury
Social skills training, 76
Sorrow, 85
Spasticity, 17
Spatial reasoning problems, 66
Special education. *See also* Educators; School reentry; Schools
evaluation and modification of the school environment, 51–52
family's reactions to, 88–89
IEP planning, 53–54
school calendar and daily scheduling, 52–53
for traumatic brain injury, 2
traumatic brain injury as category within, 43, 91
Sports injuries, 6
Staff. *See also* Educators
importance of, 45
skills in understanding neuropsychological findings, 65

training for, 56
training of, 46, 47, 49, 56
Stretching, effect on brain, 13
Substance abuse, 31
"Swiss cheese effect," 93

TBI. *See* Traumatic brain injury
Teachers. *See* Educators
Testing. *See* Assessment
Time-out, 76
Tracheostomy tube, 16, 17
Training, 46, 47, 49, 56, 95
Traumatic brain injury. *See also* Assessment; Families; Programming for students with traumatic brain injury; School reentry; Treatment for traumatic brain injury
  academic effects of, 23–24
  age influence on, 10
  assessment of, 59–66
  behavior abnormalities due to, 17
  behavioral/emotional effects of, 22–23
  bibliography on, 97–99
  causes of, 6
  cognitive effects of, 20–21
  coma due to, 15–16
  community responses to, 79
  compared with learning disabilities, 2, 94
  definition of, 1
  developmental aspects of, 9–11
  disruption of social development and, 10–11
  early acute phase of, 15–17
  effects of, 91, 93
  glossary on, 125–128
  incidence of, 3, 5
  interaction of problems resulting from, 24–25
  language effects of, 21–22
  legislation concerning, 1
  medical problems due to, 16–17
  memory disorders due to, 17
  mild brain injuries, 5
  moderate brain injuries, 5
  motor problems due to, 17
  neuropathology of, 13–14
  ongoing brain development and, 9–10
  persisting effects of, 18–24
  physical effects of, 13–25
  posttraumatic amnesia due to, 16
  programming for students with, 69–81
  psychosocial effects of, 27–32
  risk factors for, 6–7
  sensory effects of, 20
  severe brain injuries, 6
  severity of, 5–6
  treatment for, 35–41
Treatment for traumatic brain injury
  acute care phase, 35, 38–39
  components of comprehensive program, 35–38
  financing issues, 40–41
  outpatient rehabilitation, 36
  postacute care, 36
  school interactions with hospitals, 38–39
  school reentry, 36, 38

Ventricles of brain, 15
Vision problems
  as effect of traumatic brain injury, 20
  programming for, 72
Vocational rehabilitation, 80

Wechsler Adult Intelligence Scale-Revised, 62
Wechsler Intelligence Scale for Children–Revised, 62